IMAGES
of America

ELOISE

POORHOUSE, FARM, ASYLUM, AND HOSPITAL

1839–1984

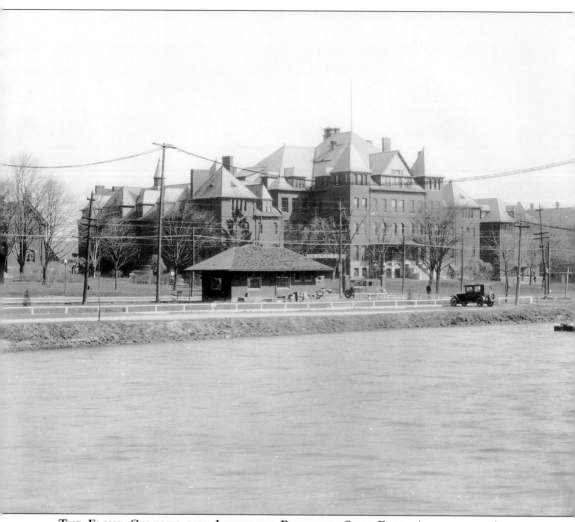

The Eloise Complex and Infirmary Building, Seen From Across the Artificial Lake, c. 1930s.

IMAGES
of America

ELOISE

POORHOUSE, FARM, ASYLUM, AND HOSPITAL

1839–1984

Patricia Ibbotson

ARCADIA
PUBLISHING

Published by Arcadia Publishing
Charleston SC, Chicago IL, Portsmouth NH, San Francisco CA

Printed in the United States of America

Library of Congress Catalog Card Number: 2002100064

For all general information contact Arcadia Publishing at:
Telephone 843-853-2070
Fax 843-853-0044
E-mail sales@arcadiapublishing.com
For customer service and orders:
Toll-Free 1-888-313-2665

Visit us on the Internet at www.arcadiapublishing.com

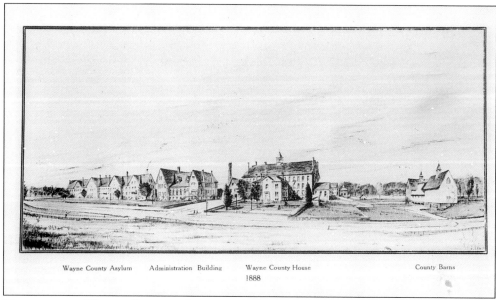

VIEW OF THE WAYNE COUNTY ASYLUM, ADMINISTRATION BUILDING, WAYNE COUNTY HOUSE (THE POORHOUSE) AND THE COUNTY BARNS IN 1888.

CONTENTS

ACKNOWLEDGMENTS

This book was made possible by the efforts of many people associated with the Friends of Eloise. It became reality due to the vision, perseverance, and dedication of Jo Johnson, currently vice president of both the Friends of Eloise and the Westland Historical Commission.

Most of the photographs are from the Eloise Museum and the Westland Historical Commission. Several are from the Walter P. Reuther Library, Wayne State University, and the Burton Historical Collection of the Detroit Public Library.

Much of the information for the captions is from *The History of Eloise* by Stanislas M. Keenan, published in Detroit by Thos. Smith Press in 1913. *A History of the Wayne County Infirmary, Psychiatric, and General Hospital Complex at Eloise, Michigan 1832–1982* by Alvin C. Clark was also used as a reference in compiling the information. Extensive use was also made of the annual reports of the Superintendents of the Poor, later called the Wayne County Board of County Institutions. Information concerning the buildings and the people of Eloise also came from interviews with former employees and people who lived on the Eloise grounds, including Betty Zimmerman, Frances Hancock, E.J. Conklin, M.D., Edward Missavage, M.D., Bert Randall, and Jane Hudson Woodrow. They also donated some of the photographs used in this book.

INTRODUCTION

Eloise derived its name from its post office. The post office was established in 1894 and named after the postmaster of Detroit's four-year old daughter, Eloise. Although this institution had several other official names over the years, among them the Wayne County Poorhouse, The Wayne County House, and Wayne County General Hospital and Infirmary, the name Eloise was the one most commonly associated with this complex. It became a generic term used to designate the complex and all the buildings in it. And, although this complex was a poorhouse, a large farm, a tuberculosis sanitarium, an infirmary and a major general hospital, most people associate it as being only a mental asylum. There are many people in the area that had connections with Eloise or had relatives who were patients there. Local interest in the "ghosts of Eloise" has also been strong and there have been ghostly expeditions to the grounds in search of these spirits.

It all started when the Wayne County Poor House was founded in 1832. It was located at Gratiot and Mt. Elliott Avenues in Hamtramck Township, 2 miles from the Detroit city limits. By 1834 this poorhouse was already in a very bad condition, so 280 acres were purchased in Nankin Township, which is now the City of Westland. The property belonged to Samuel and Nancy Torbert and Samuel's father. The Black Horse Tavern, which served as a stagecoach stop between Detroit and Chicago on what was then the Old Chicago Road, was located on this property. In those days it was a two-day ride by stagecoach from Hamtramck Township to Nankin Township. In April of 1839, 35 persons were transferred from the poorhouse in Hamtramck Township to the new one in Nankin Township; 111 refused to go to the "awful wilderness."

Eloise evolved into a self-supporting community with its own police and fire department, railroad and trolley stations, bakery, amusement hall, laundries, and a powerhouse. It even had a schoolhouse that was used for about ten years. In addition, there were many farm buildings, including barns, a piggery, root cellars, a tobacco curing building, and greenhouses. All of the buildings housing patients were given an alphabetical designation, starting with "A" building and ending with "P" building. As buildings were remodeled or torn down, these designations changed so that the same building could be known as "B" Building and later "E" Building. There was also low rent housing for employees and about 20 percent of the staff lived on the grounds. It was not uncommon for someone to meet his future spouse while working at Eloise and many children grew up on the grounds. Many lasting friendships were also formed among the staff, patients, and area residents.

As the years went on, the institution grew larger and larger, a reflection in the increases in the population in the Detroit area. From only 35 residents on 280 acres in 1839, the complex grew dramatically after the Civil War until the total land involved was 902 acres and the total number of patients was about 10,000. One building alone, "N" Building or Kelley Hall, constructed in four months in 1930, could house 7,000 patients. One measurement the size of Eloise is in the statistics of deaths. Between February 1, 1944 and 1949, there were 8,291 deaths at the Wayne County General Hospital and Infirmary; 533 of these patients are buried in the Eloise Cemetery in numbered graves.

The population peaked during the Great Depression and then began to decrease. The farm operations ceased in 1958 and the complex began purchasing all its food. Some of the large psychiatric buildings were vacated in 1973. The large hospital complex started closing in 1977 when the State of Michigan took over the psychiatric division. The general hospital was closed in 1984. The buildings sat vacant for years and were subjected to vandalism. Wayne County then demolished all but a few of the old buildings.

Today the land that once was Eloise has been developed into a strip mall, a golf course, and condominiums. There is only one building currently in use. It is "D" Building or the Kay Beard Building located at 30712 Michigan Avenue in Westland, Michigan. Kay Beard is a Wayne County Commissioner who tried to prevent the closure of the institution. At one time this was the administration building, and it also was used for psychiatric admissions. It also housed the post office. Today there is a small museum here. Frank Rembisz, the Director of the Office on Aging for the County of Wayne and unofficial County historian, collected artifacts and started the museum. The Friends of Eloise are now assisting in preserving the memorabilia and memories of Eloise.

One

POORHOUSE, FARM, ASYLUM

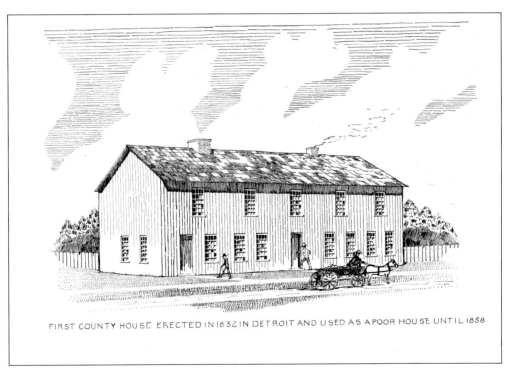

FIRST COUNTY HOUSE ERECTED IN 1832 IN DETROIT AND USED AS A POOR HOUSE UNTIL 1838

THE FIRST POORHOUSE, 1832–1838. This ramshackle building was located on part of the Leib farm at Gratiot and Mt. Elliott streets in Detroit. The cholera epidemic of 1834 caused over 50 children to be made orphans and many were sent to the poorhouse. In 1837, there were 80–100 inmates in the poorhouse. More space was needed, but land was expensive in the city so a move was made to the country.

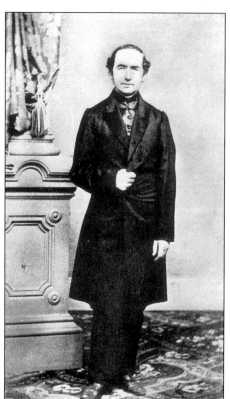

THE REVEREND MARTIN KUNDIG. Kundig was a noted Detroit clergyman and humanitarian. Known for his heroic work during the cholera epidemic, he was also the first commissioner of the poor. He did not limit his expenditures to the small amount he was allotted by the County, but spent his own monies on the poor. As a result, he went into debt and his personal property was seized and sold at auction. Fr. Kundig left Detroit for Milwaukee in 1842 and later repaid all his Detroit debts.

THE BLACK HORSE TAVERN, 1828. This wooden log cabin and land were purchased in February 1839 for $800. The tavern was run by Samuel S. and Nancy Torbert. The Detroit and Ypsilanti four-horse stage stopped here on its daily trips to allow passengers a short rest. Tales were told of whisky sold at 15¢ a gallon and a free-for-all fight an hourly occurrence at the Black Horse Tavern. This site was in Nankin Township 16 miles from Detroit.

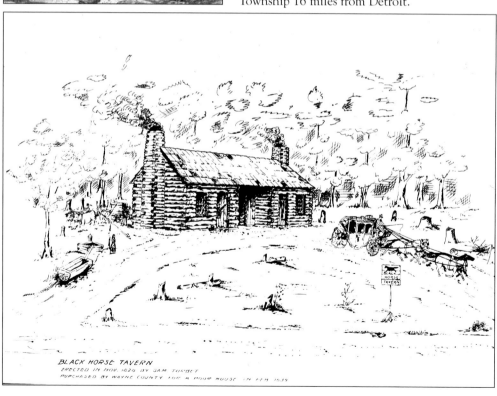

BLACK HORSE TAVERN
ERECTED IN NOV. 1828 BY SAM TORBERT
PURCHASED BY WAYNE COUNTY FOR A POOR HOUSE IN FEB. 1839

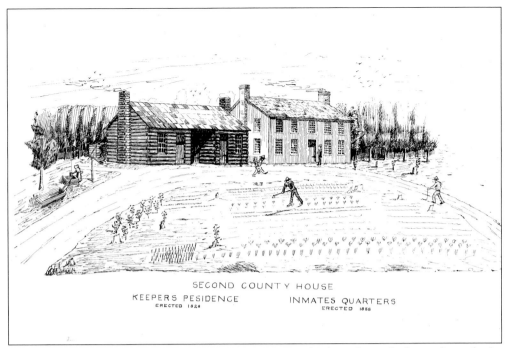

THE SECOND POORHOUSE OR COUNTY HOUSE, 1838. The log cabin, which was formerly the Black Horse Tavern, became the keeper's quarters and in 1838-39 a frame building was put up to house the inmates. A frame cookhouse was erected in back of the log building and was used for cooking for both inmates and the keeper's family.

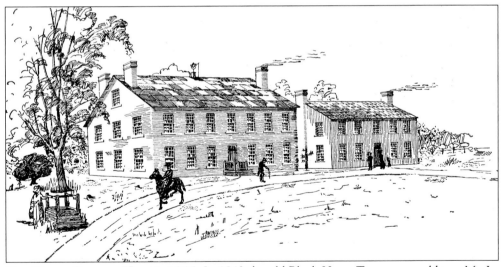

THE THIRD COUNTY HOUSE, 1845. In 1843 the old Black Horse Tavern was sold to a Mr. La Platt for the princely sum of $2. This new brick building built on the site housed the keeper and his family and the old and feeble inmates. Other inmates were housed in the frame building. A portion of the basement of the new brick building was used to house drunks and unruly inmates and chains were fastened to the walls.

11

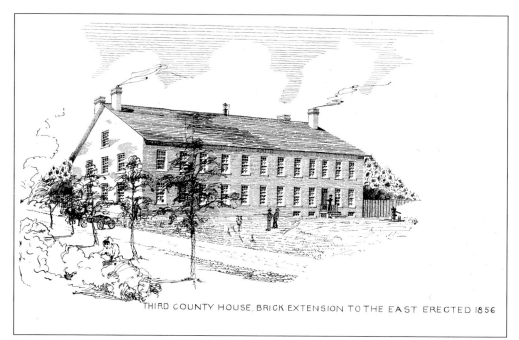

THIRD COUNTY HOUSE, BRICK EXTENSION TO THE EAST ERECTED 1856

EXTENSION OF THIRD COUNTY HOUSE, 1856. Ten years after the third county house was built, more space was needed, so this brick extension to the east was added in 1856. It had a finished basement with a dining room, bakery and furnace room and was surrounded by a whitewashed fence. A vegetable garden and cherry orchard were in front.

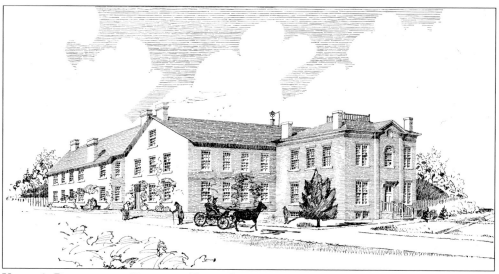

KEEPER'S RESIDENCE IN FRONT OF THIRD COUNTY HOUSE, 1865. A.L. Chase, the keeper at the time, was the first to occupy this addition. In addition to housing the keeper, the building provided an office and storeroom for the clerk, and a room for the Superintendents of the Poor to meet. There was also a bedroom that was used by the resident physician in later years.

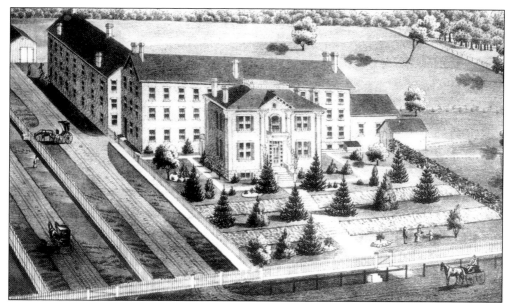

COUNTY ASYLUM AND POORHOUSE, 1876. A bird's-eye view of the Third County House after the main building and wings were raised to three stories. The drawing is from H. Belden & Co.'s *Wayne County Atlas*.

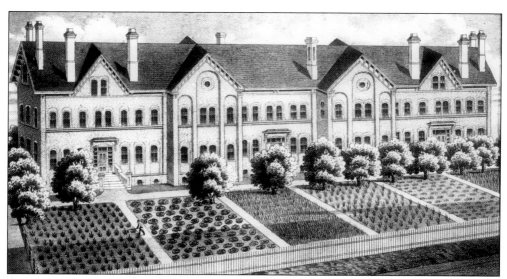

ANOTHER VIEW OF THE COUNTY ASYLUM AND POORHOUSE, 1876. This drawing also appeared in H. Belden & Co.'s *Wayne County Atlas*. The center of the building was erected in 1868 and the wings in 1876.

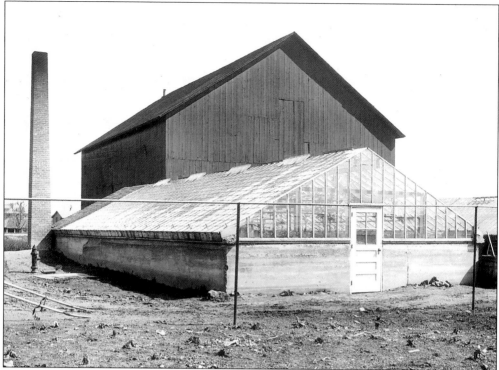

FARM GREENHOUSE, 1917. A farm was kept from 1839 on to feed the inmates. The first crops grown were peas, corn, oats, onions, beets, rutabagas, and pickles. The farm expanded as the population increased. The farm greenhouse enabled the hospital to advance the growing season three to four weeks in the growing of crops. The frame barn in the rear was erected in 1876.

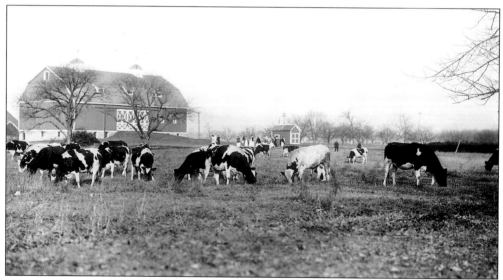

VIEW OF HOLSTEIN-FRIESIAN HERD, 1912. In 1898 eight cows and bulls of the Holstein-Fresian breed were purchased to produce wholesome milk economically for the patients of Eloise. This herd quickly grew in size to over 100 by 1917 and some were exhibited at the Michigan State Fair. The grain barn, built in 1875, and other farm buildings are in seen the background.

14

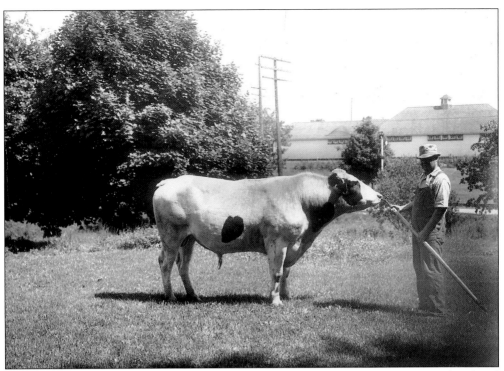

DUTCHLAND WINANA SIR ASCALON NO. 126990, 1915. This bull shown with a farm hand was the herd sire.

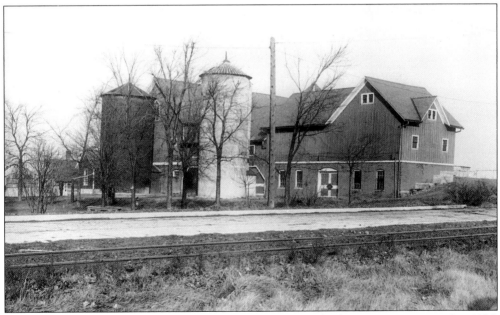

DAIRY BARN, C. 1915. Formerly known as the County Barn, the first section was erected in 1896. The building was torn down in 1925. This photo, as are many of the others of the same time period, is by Manning Bros., Commercial Photographers, 22–24 Witherell St., Detroit, Michigan.

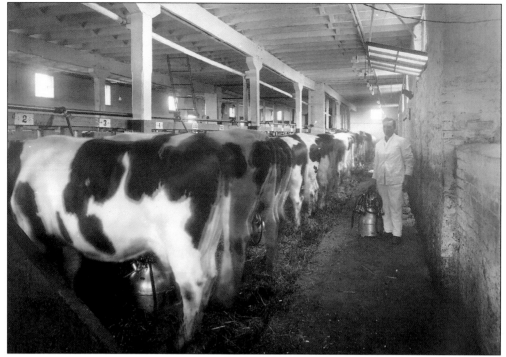

DAIRY ROOM AND ELECTRIC MILKER, 1915. The dairy barn was equipped with electric milkers, cooling devices and all the other modern conveniences of the time. Attached to the eastside of the dairy barn was a milk house. The milk was put in bottles marked *Eloise* or *Wayne County Hospital.*

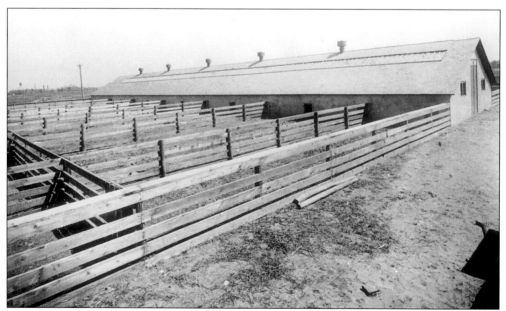

THE PIGGERY. The raising of hogs was carried on from the beginning. The original piggery building was erected in 1889. This building was erected south of Michigan Avenue in 1917. The raising of hogs for both food for the inmates and for the market proved to be a profitable enterprise.

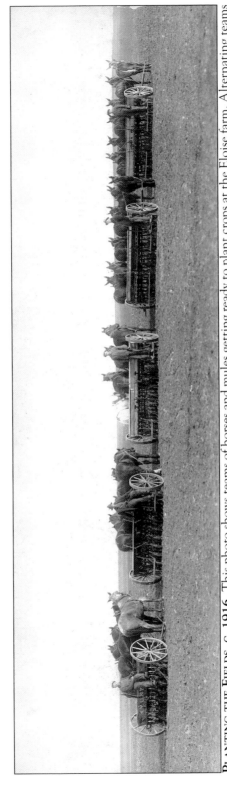

PLANTING THE FIELDS, C. 1916. This photo shows teams of horses and mules getting ready to plant crops at the Eloise farm. Alternating teams drilled and seeded. Inmates were paid 50¢ a day for working on the farm. The total cost of wages for the inmates in 1916 was $3,000.

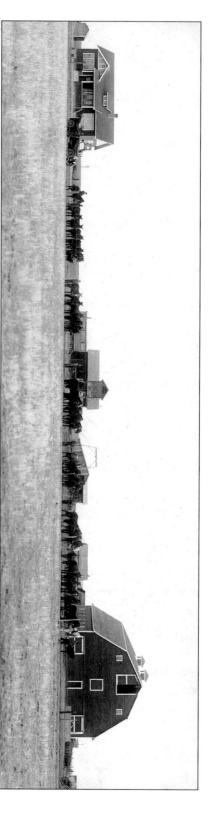

VIEW OF THE ELOISE FARM, C. 1916. Farm hands pose with their teams of horses and mules in front of the farm buildings. The farm foreman was Thomas Burt. In 1916 the farm production included, among other produce, 6,442 heads of cabbage, 3,006 muskmelons, and 3,187 quarts of strawberries.

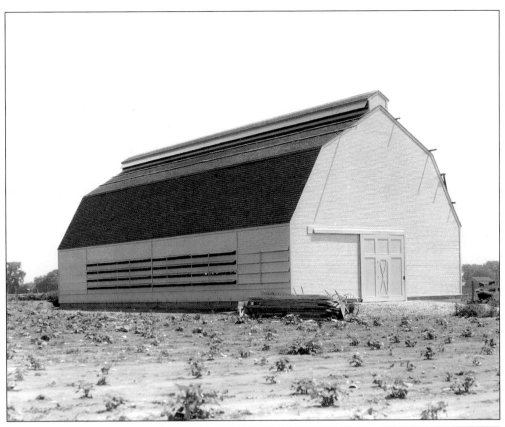

TOBACCO CURING BUILDING, 1936. The harvesting of tobacco crops began in 1933 and a drying shed was put up. This building was constructed in 1936. It was located south of Michigan Avenue next to the piggery.

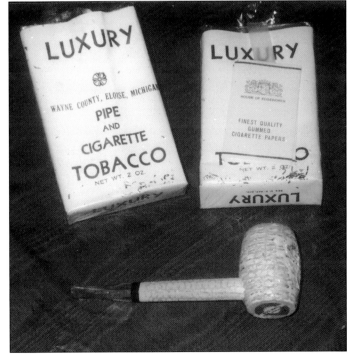

TOBACCO SUPPLIES. The tobacco was packaged for roll-your-own cigarettes in packages marked *Eloise*. Many of the patients smoked cigarettes at the time or used corncob pipes furnished by the institution. These items can be viewed at the Eloise Museum.

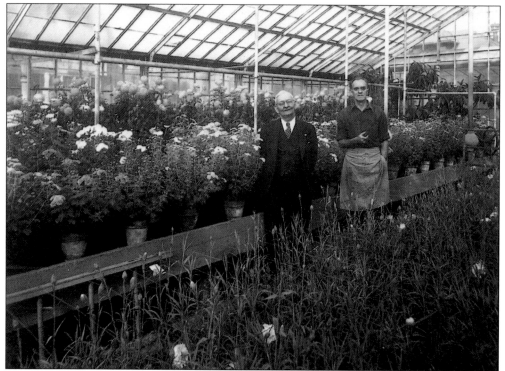

KEEPERS OF THE ELOISE GREENHOUSES, 1940S. The Hudsons—Charles, the father and Jack, the son—both gardeners, are seen in one of the two Eloise greenhouses. The floral greenhouse supplied beautiful flowers to the grounds and holiday flowers, such as Easter lilies, for the buildings. Eloise was known for its landscaped grounds.

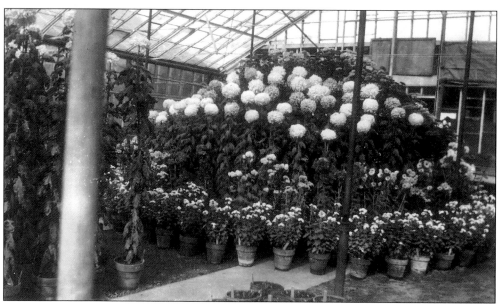

BEAUTIFUL MUMS, 1940S. The Hudson's photographed these beautiful giant mums in the floral greenhouse.

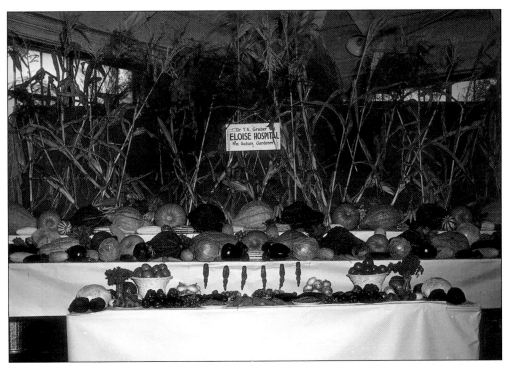

DISPLAY AT THE STATE FAIR, 1940S. This bountiful harvest from the 500-acre Eloise farm was part of a display at the Michigan State Fair.

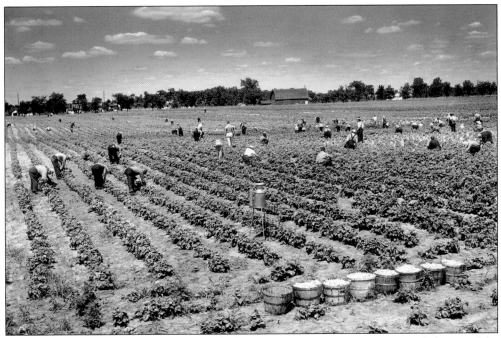

WORKING IN THE FIELDS, 1940S. From the beginning patients or inmates provided most of the labor in planting and harvesting the crops. Here they are harvesting yellow beans, but tobacco is growing in the foreground.

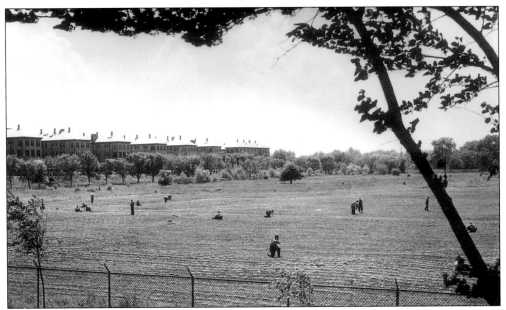

ANOTHER VIEW OF PATIENTS WORKING IN THE FIELDS, 1940S. This section of the County Farm was on the north side of Michigan Avenue as viewed from Henry Ruff Road. The rears of several psychiatric buildings can be seen in the background.

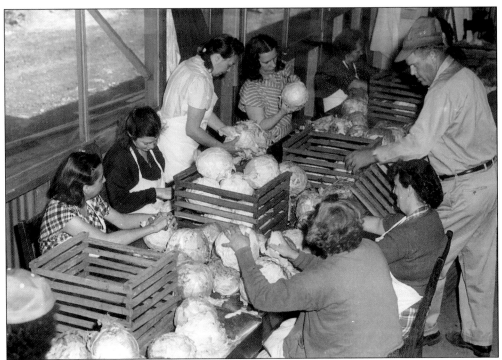

THE CANNERY, 1952. One paid employee was in charge of 75 patients. These patients are shown making sauerkraut. The cannery was built in 1939. It was located just south of the railroad tracks next to the slaughterhouse. Sixty-five tons a month of fruit and vegetables were processed with help from the patients. The cannery was phased out in 1971.

Two

PSYCHIATRIC DIVISION

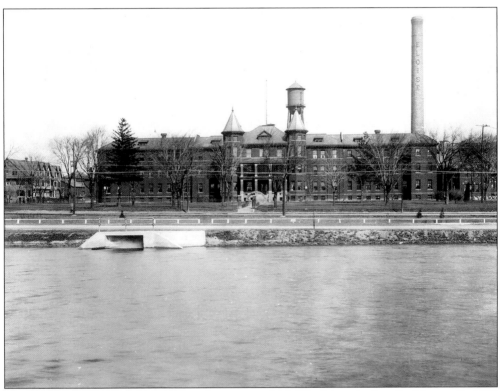

PANORAMIC VIEW OF THE HOSPITAL COMPLEX, 1925. The Main Asylum Building, called "B" Building, then "E" Building, is shown across the artificial lake. The center of this building had been reconstructed from an existing building in 1899. The east wing of the building was erected in 1904 and the west wing in 1905. It was razed in 1955. Behind "E" Building are a water tower and the power plant smokestack. To the left of the asylum is the Apartment Building and Cafeteria that was built in 1921.

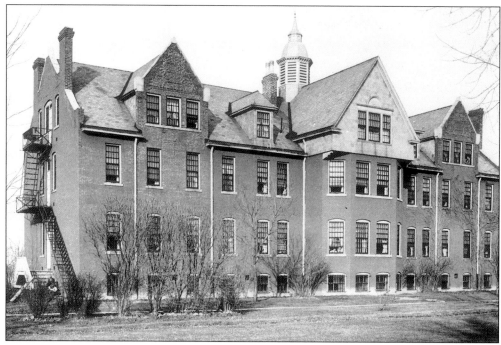

"F" BUILDING, 1893. This was also called the Woman's New Building when it was first built. It was used to house a "better class" of the female insane. Keenan considered it to be one of the best on the hospital grounds. In 1932, when all the buildings were given new alphabetical designations, the building became "C" Building. It was razed in 1955.

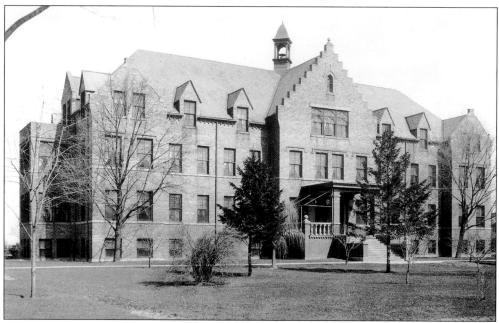

"D" BUILDING, C. 1920. This was first called the Women's Insane Hospital when it was built in 1903. There were sun porches for the patients on each floor. It provided housing for 125 patients and 8 attendants. It was renamed "G" Building in 1932. It was razed in 1955.

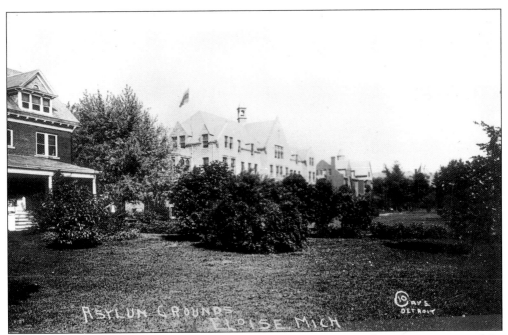

ELOISE POSTCARD, 1916. In this rare early view of the asylum grounds, one can see part of the double residence to the left and "D" Building to the right. This postcard was sent by Bernard Doyle of Wayne to Mr. H. Bamber of Highland, Michigan. (Courtesy of the Burton Historical Collection of the Detroit Public Library.)

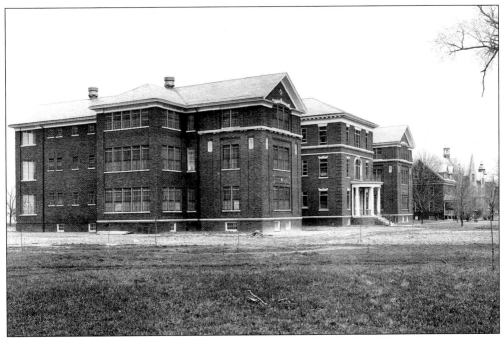

"E" BUILDING, 1915. Built in 1915, this building, which housed female psychiatric patients, was partially destroyed by fire on March 27, 1923. It was renamed "H" Building in 1932 and was vacated in 1973.

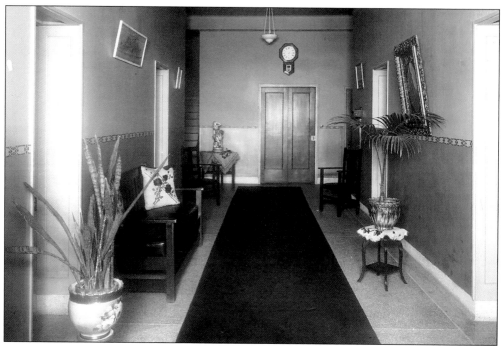

INTERIOR OF "E" BUILDING, 1915. The main corridor of the building created a home-like welcome. The building was designed to be light and airy with light gray trim and a wainscoting of darker gray with a stenciled finish. All the corners of the walls were rounded or beveled to prevent dust settling.

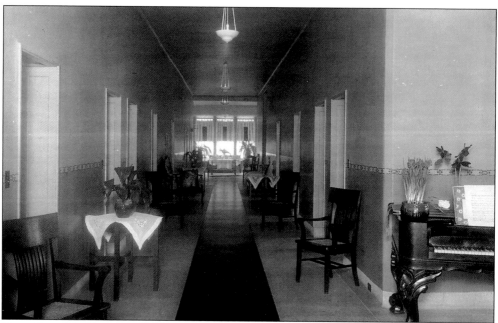

EAST CORRIDOR, BUILDING "E," 1915. Note the fine piano to the right. All the floors were marble terrazzo. This building also had the first metal window frames. "E" building was called the "most pretentious, handsomest and best equipped building at Eloise" when it was new.

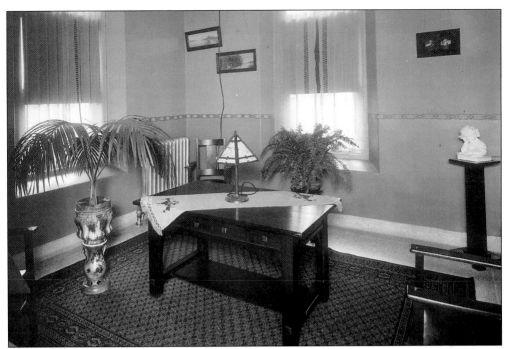

RECEPTION ROOM OF "E" BUILDING, 1915. This looks more like the lobby of a charming hotel than the entrance to a mental institution.

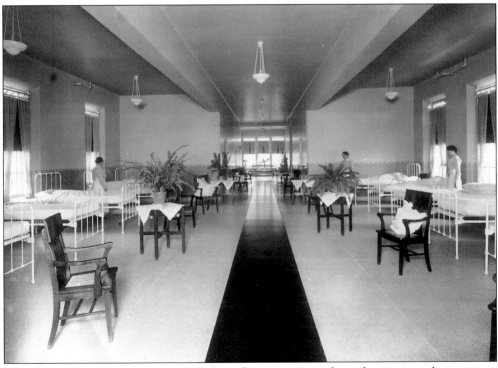

LADIES WARD "E" BUILDING, 1915. Attendants are pictured standing next to their patients in this spacious ward.

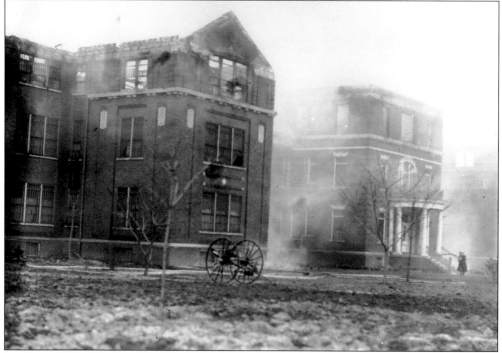

AFTERMATH OF FIRE IN "E" BUILDING, 1923. The fire made the front page of *The Detroit News* on March 28, 1923. Two patients were killed in the fire. Almost all the people residing within a mile of the hospital fought the fire with the firefighters or helped in the rescue work. The building was insured for $170,000 and it was reconstructed in 1923-24. (Courtesy of the Walter P. Reuther Library, Wayne State University.)

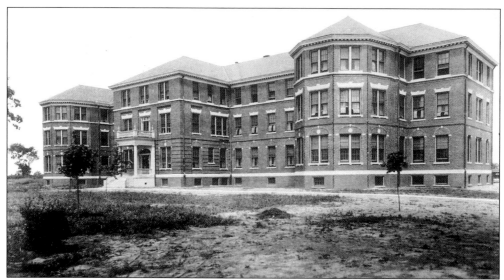

"F" BUILDING, 1921. This psychiatric hospital building, later called "I" building, was built at the beginning of the big expansion of the Eloise complex. It was completed in 1921 and was located on the corner of Michigan Avenue and Merriman Road. It was used to house 240 female patients and was vacated in 1973.

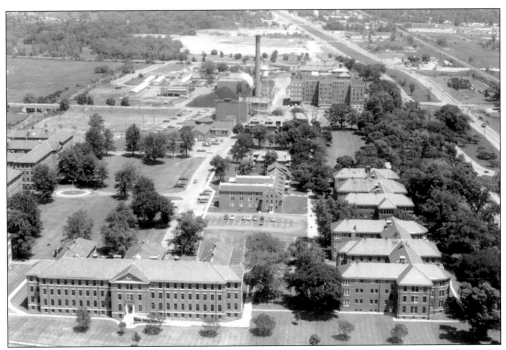

AERIAL VIEW OF "J" BUILDING. This photo shows part of the Eloise grounds from the perspective of Merriman Road with "J" building in the front facing the camera. It was built in 1924 and was one of eight buildings that housed female psychiatric patients. It was vacated in 1973 and used as the Wayne County Office on Aging until it was demolished.

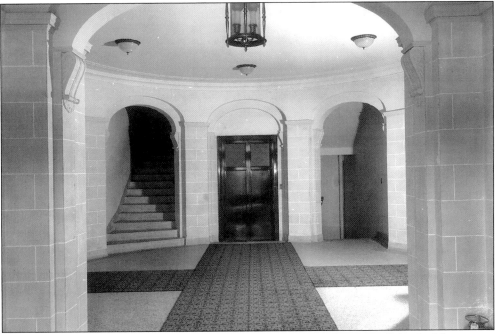

VIEW OF LOBBY OF "J" BUILDING, 1924. The interiors of many of the buildings were architectural gems. The materials used and the workmanship could not be duplicated today.

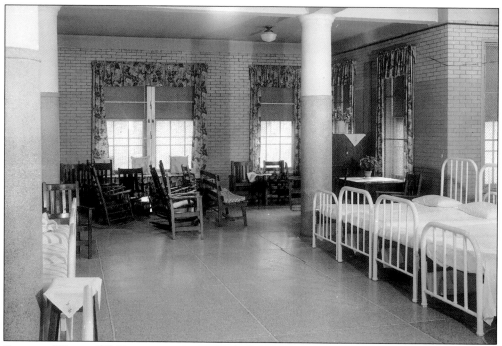

PATIENT WARD, "J" BUILDING, 1924. Each dormitory style ward had an area where patients could sit during the day. Many of the patients were elderly and enjoyed the rocking chairs.

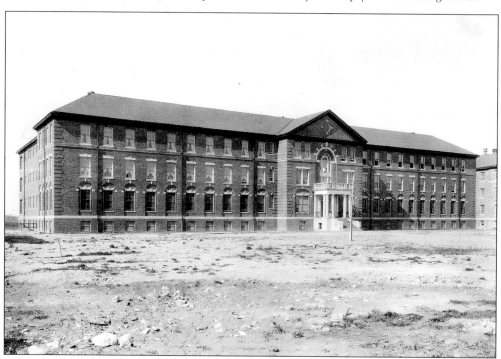

"I" BUILDING, 1928. "I" building later became "L" Building and is in several other photos in this book. The administrative and nurses' quarters occupied the south side of the center section of the first, second, and third floors. It was vacated in 1973.

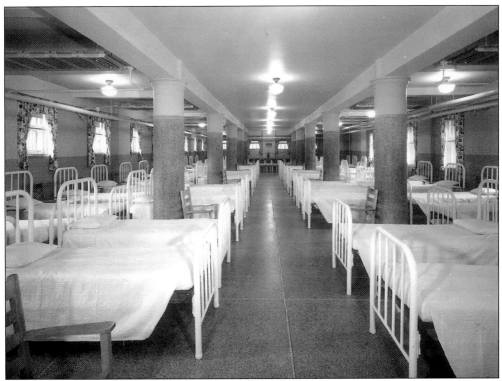

PATIENT WARD, "L" BUILDING. L-1 was located in the basement and was used to house female psychiatric patients.

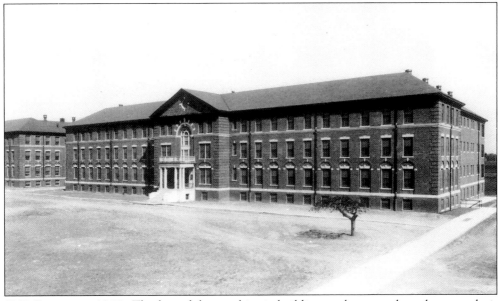

"M" BUILDING, 1929. The last of the psychiatric buildings to be erected on the grounds, it was used to house both men and women psychiatric patients who had tuberculosis. Later it was used for male psychiatric patients. After the psychiatric division closed, it was used as a Wayne County Jail Annex for a short time.

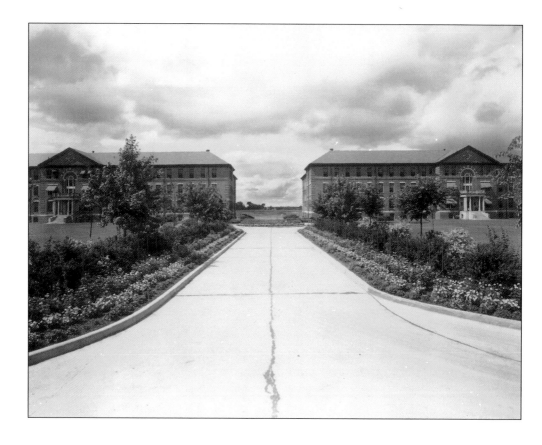

FLORAL DRIVEWAY AND ROSE GARDEN, 1930S. A road that ended in a circular drive separated "L" and "M" Building. The grounds were carefully landscaped as evidenced by this photo. Below is Charles Hudson, one of the gardeners, posing in front of some of his handiwork.

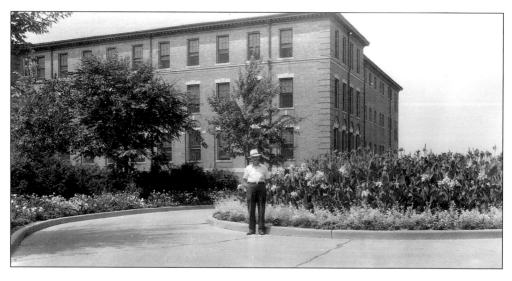

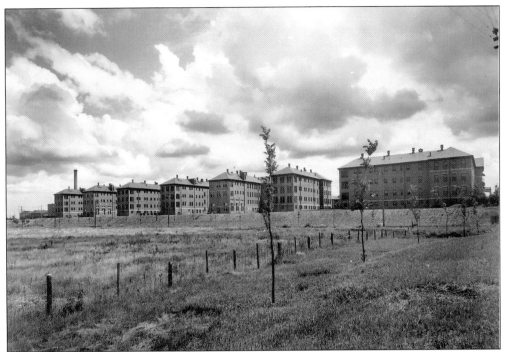

REAR VIEW OF PSYCHIATRIC HOSPITAL BUILDINGS, 1930S. From left to right are "M," "L," and "K" Buildings. The view from Merriman Road shows the large wings on the back of the buildings and gives a better perspective of the size of the psychiatric buildings.

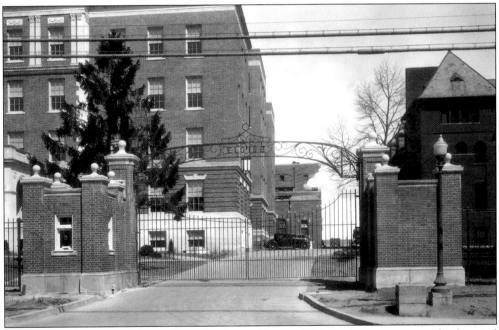

THE SIGN ABOVE THE GATE SAYS IT ALL—ELOISE. This is the entrance to the hospital complex in the 1930s, with a guardhouse to the left of the gate. On the left is "D" Building, and to the right is the William J. Seymour Hospital.

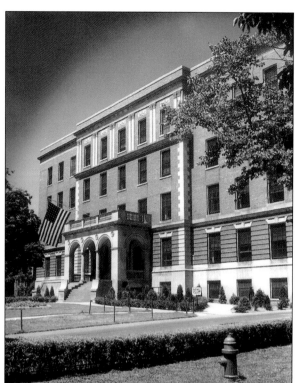

PSYCHIATRIC ADMISSION CENTER, 1950S. "D" Building, built in 1931, is now the Kay Beard Building. It was first used to house the administrative offices of the institution, the post office, and the admitting and treatment wards. In addition to patient wards, there were two complete apartments for employees on the third and fourth floors and rooms for housing attendants. Only the first two floors are still in use, currently housing the Wayne County Office on Aging and the Head Start program.

ENTRANCE TO "D" BUILDING, 1931. The granite steps and stone porch are shown along with the new landscaping when the building first opened. The style is Georgian colonial.

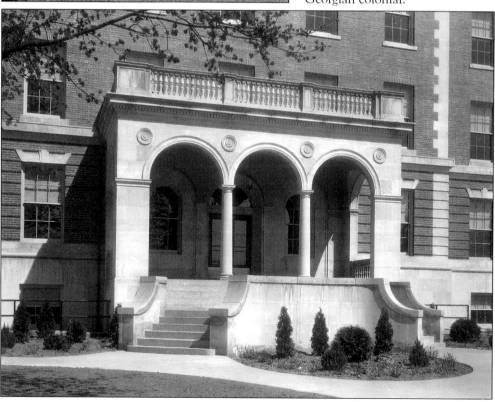

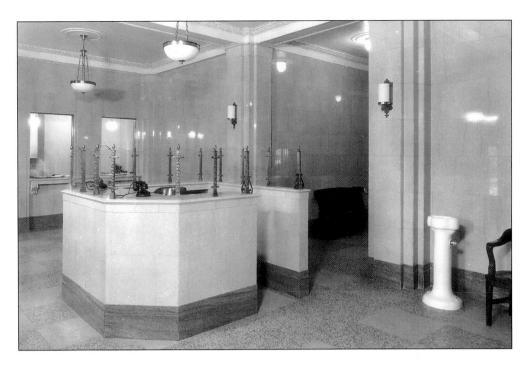

INFORMATION BOOTH AND LOBBY, "D" BUILDING, 1931. These two views show the building as it looked when it was new. The walls and columns are of travernelle Tennessee marble and the floor is squared terrazzo. To the left of the waiting room was the office of the superintendent and the boardroom. To the right were the post office and the offices of the bookkeeping department.

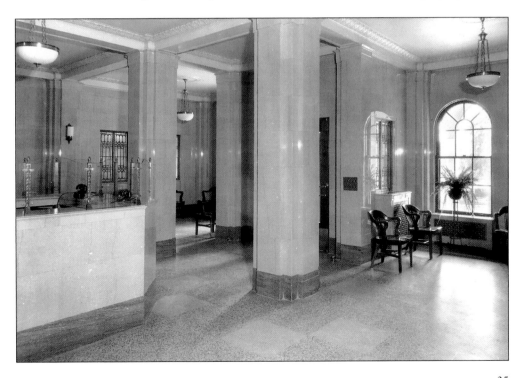

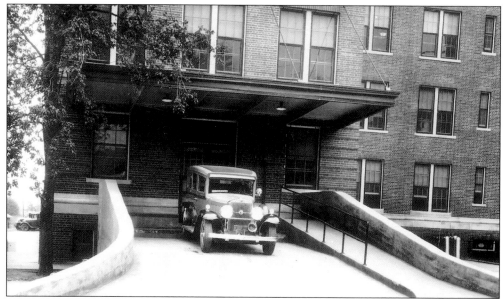

AMBULANCE ENTRANCE AND LOADING DOCK, 1930S. Here is where patients and supplies were brought to "D" building. This view of "D" Building is essentially unchanged today.

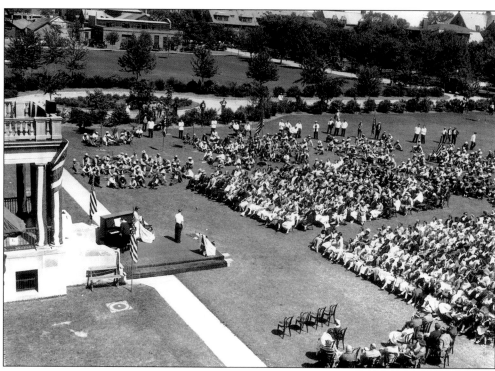

A PATIENT PAGEANT, 1936. Two-hundred and fifty psychiatric patients took part in a pageant, which was put on in front of "L" Building in June of 1936. Approximately 1,000 patients were in the audience. This was part of the occupational therapy program directed by Mrs. Myrtle Martin. The laundry building can be seen in the background. (Courtesy of the Walter P. Reuther Library, Wayne State University.)

A LOCKED WARD, 1939. Employee Ruth Brooks opens the door for a patient.

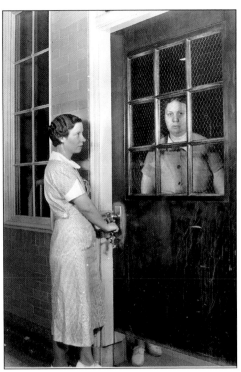

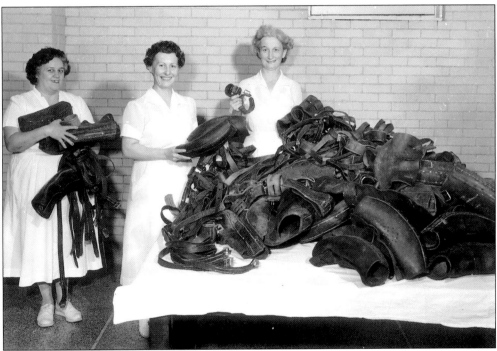

LEATHER RESTRAINTS, 1940S. Attendants display a pile of restraints that were used on psychiatric patients. In the days before Prozac and other drugs that control psychiatric symptoms, patients were controlled with leather restraints and strait jackets. In addition to restraints, "quiet rooms" or seclusion rooms were used for combative or loud patients.

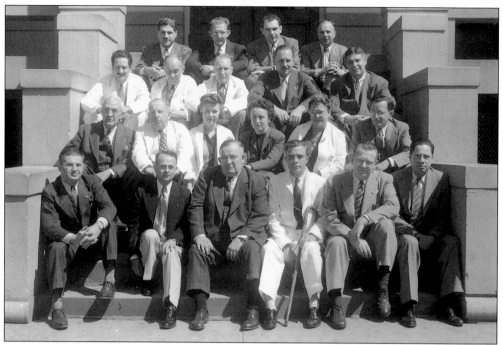

PSYCHIATRIC STAFF, JUNE 1946. They are, from left to right: (front row) Drs. L.S. Lipshutz, Ira M. Altshuler, T.K. Gruber, Milton Erickson, and Edward Hinko; (second row) Roland Athay, Walter Squires, Natalia Janicki, Eva Beck, and Rudolph Leiser; (third row) Ben Jeffries, James K. Linton, next two unidentified, and Burton Schmeir; (back row) Anthony Abruzzo, John "Jack" Belisle, Joseph Slusky, and Morris Golden.

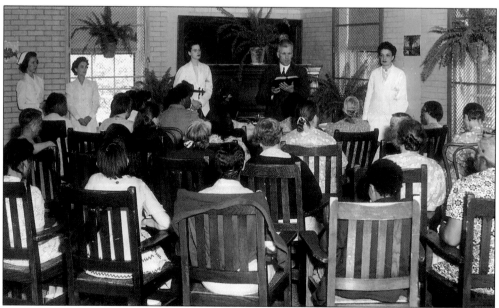

DEVOTIONAL SERVICES, 1946. Religious services were conducted for patients on both the wards and in the auditorium chapels. Shown in this photo are Mary Earl, Avis Newcomb, an unidentified minister, Winifred Salommer Kemp Reel, and Jane Matney, the music therapist.

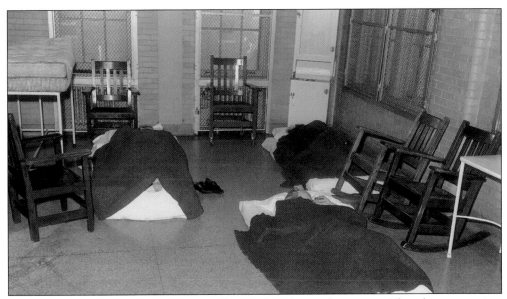

SLEEPING ON THE SUN PORCHES, 1947. The number of mental patients at Eloise kept increasing. Ward N-106 of the Infirmary building was converted to use for 400 mental patients in 1943. The State of Michigan had no vacant beds to relieve the overcrowding at Eloise. By 1946 the mental patients numbered 4,300 and there weren't enough beds, so these women had to sleep on the floor of the sun porch. (Courtesy of the Walter P. Reuther Library, Wayne State University.)

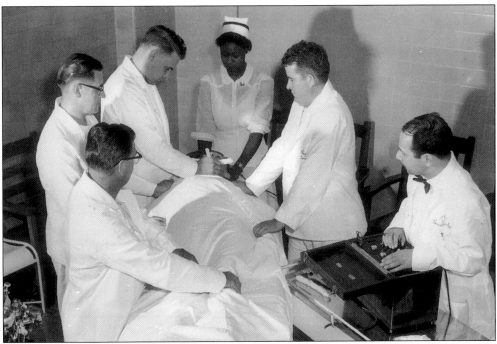

ELECTROSHOCK THERAPY, 1952. E.S.T. was used on patients suffering from several types of mental illness. A physician and nurse made home visits to perform this treatment on wealthier patients whose families did not want the stigma of being treated at Eloise. This treatment is now back in vogue for the treatment of depression. Dr. Ralph Green is at the E.S.T. machine.

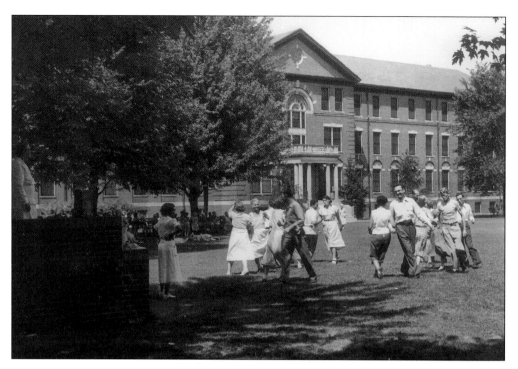

RECREATIONAL THERAPY, 1946. Patients engaged in recreational therapy on the Eloise grounds. This was one of many techniques used in treating mental illness and is still a treatment method used today. The prescribed use of recreational activities improves the functional living competence of persons with physical, mental, emotional and/or social disadvantages.

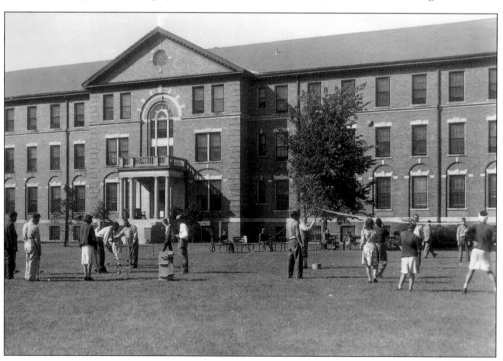

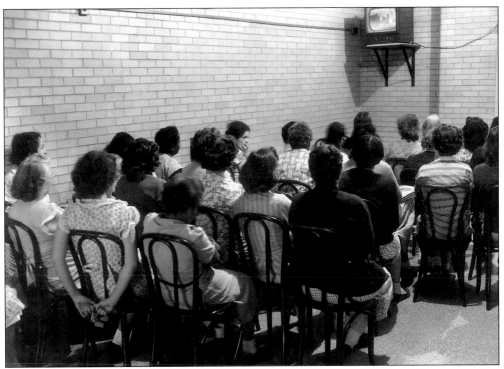

TELEVISION THERAPY, 1952. Some psychiatrists at that time thought that television was "an amazing way to treat neurotics and mild schizoids." Comedies and love stories were thought to be the most therapeutic. Even if not effective as a treatment, television provided entertainment and a way to pass the time.

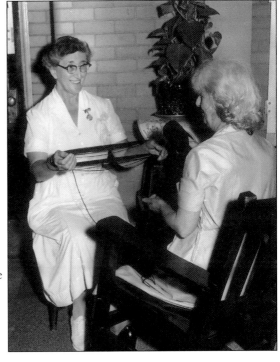

TENDING TO THEIR KNITTING, 1954. This photo, dated October 1, 1954, shows Beatrice Janchick, the chief female hospital attendant supervisor, holding yarn for a patient. Mrs. Janchick also ran an "Apparel for Milady" shop in "D" Building, which made employee-donated clothing available to female patients.

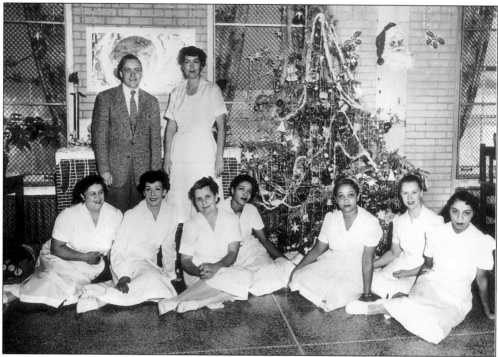

HOLIDAY PARTY, C. 1950. Here, the Hospital staff poses in front of a Christmas tree.

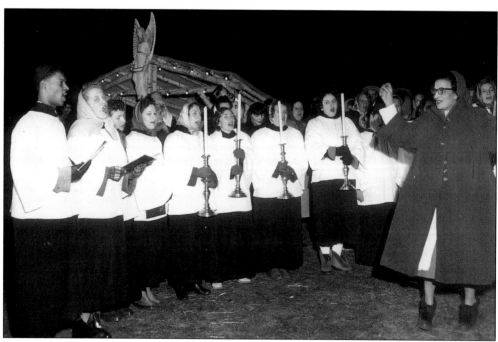

CHRISTMAS FESTIVITIES, 1955. Led by the Music Therapist, Jane Matney, a group of patients sing Christmas songs at the outdoor lighting of the Christmas tree. Music therapy was initiated at Eloise in 1937 and Michigan State University developed a degree program in this field with an internship program at Eloise.

Three

TUBERCULOSIS
SANITARIUM
AND THE GENERAL HOSPITAL AND INFIRMARY

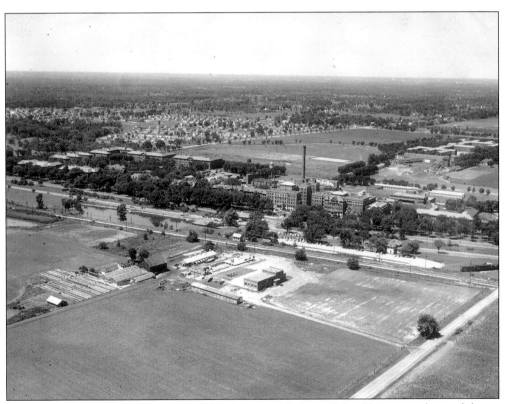

AERIAL VIEW OF ELOISE, C. 1950. This is an aerial view of the Eloise complex and farms. Today, Wayne County owns less than 30 acres on this site and most of the land was sold to the Ford Motor Company and other developers. Note the Eloise smokestack in the center of the photo, which still exists.

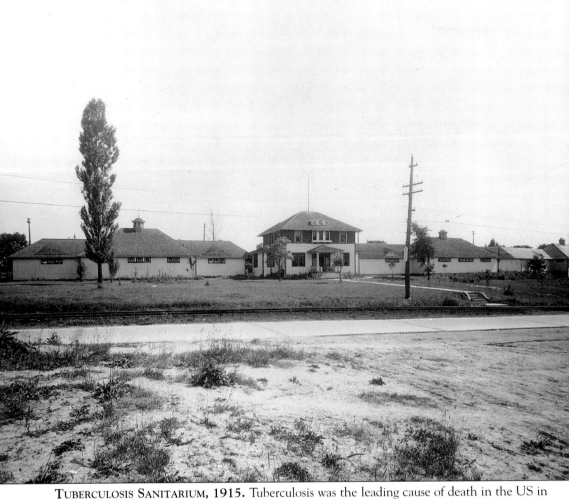

TUBERCULOSIS SANITARIUM, 1915. Tuberculosis was the leading cause of death in the US in 1903 when two tents were erected on the grounds for 24 patients. One tent was for men and the other for women. These tents were along the east side and the east wing of the County House. Patients with tuberculosis had to be isolated from other patients. The theory of the time was that fresh air and sunshine would cure tuberculosis. The number of patients with tuberculosis kept increasing, so in 1909 a more permanent structure was built. The *Eloise Sanitarium*, as it was called, was located on the south side of Michigan Avenue between the highway and the Michigan Central Railroad. The TB patients at Eloise had exhausted all other resources and were in the last stages of the disease. The TB Sanitarium was phased out in 1923.

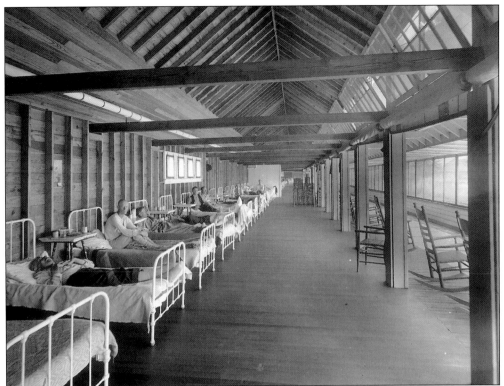

INTERIOR OF A DORMITORY, 1914. The majority of the tuberculosis patients were male, in a ratio of about ten to one. They were housed in dormitories that Keenan referred to as "shacks." There were screens and rocking chairs along one side so patients could get fresh air.

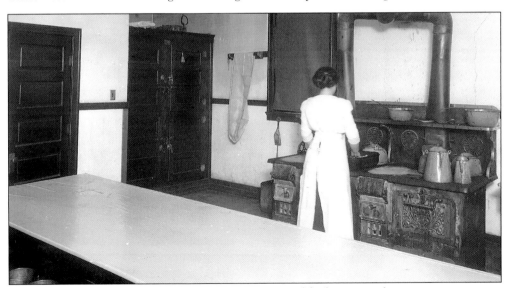

KITCHEN OF THE TB SANITARIUM, 1915. Nutrition and fresh air were the common treatments for TB at the time and meals were made under strict dietary guidelines. Nutrition, rest, and diet were the cornerstones of treatment as there were no drugs that were effective in combating this disease.

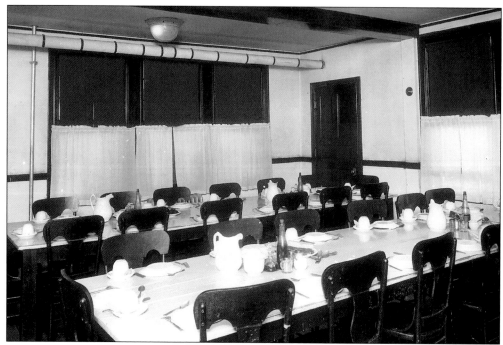

REFECTORY OR DINING ROOM OF THE TB SANITARIUM, 1915. One of the two dining rooms is shown. Extra care was taken with leftover food. Paper napkins, food, floor sweepings, etc. were incinerated. Every precaution was taken to prevent the spread of the disease.

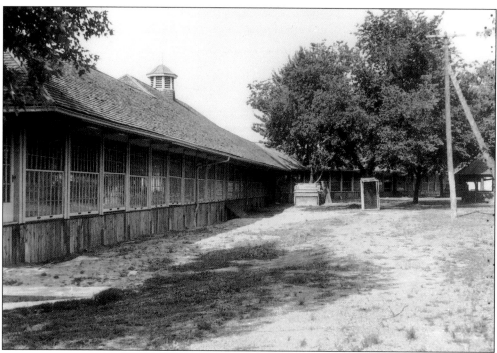

EXTERIOR OF A DORMITORY, 1931. This photo was taken after the TB Sanitarium was phased out. (Courtesy of the Walter P. Reuther Library, Wayne State University.)

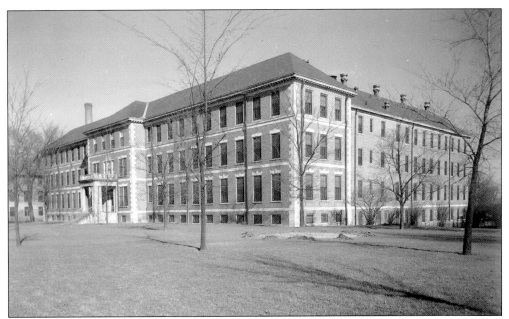

"D" Building, 1925. This was a women's infirmary building designed by Detroit architects Maul & Lentz, and it was used to house the aged and infirm. It was located at the corner of Michigan Avenue and Henry Ruff. It had a bed capacity of 392. The nurses' quarters occupied the south center section of the first, second and third floors. Its name changed to "A" Building in 1932.

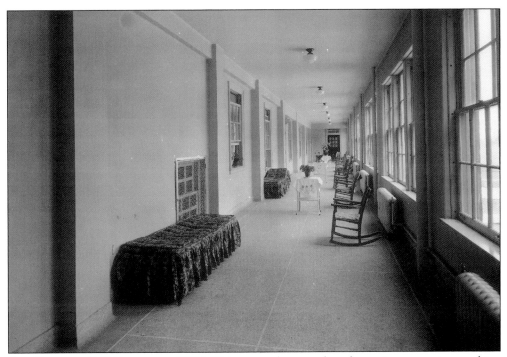

Sun Room in "D" Building, 1925. This was a pleasant place for patients to enjoy sunshine without exposure to the weather, and broke the monotony of being in the dormitory-style wards. The area was heated for year-round use.

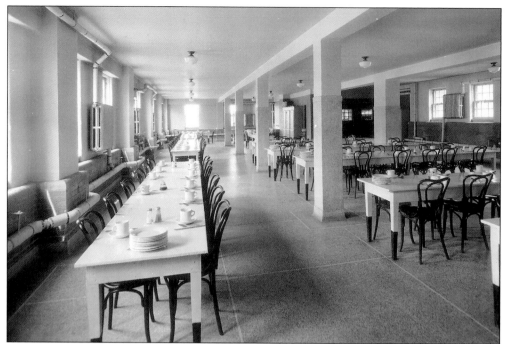

DINING ROOM IN "D" BUILDING, 1925. Patients who were able to walk had their meals in this room, which was located in the basement.

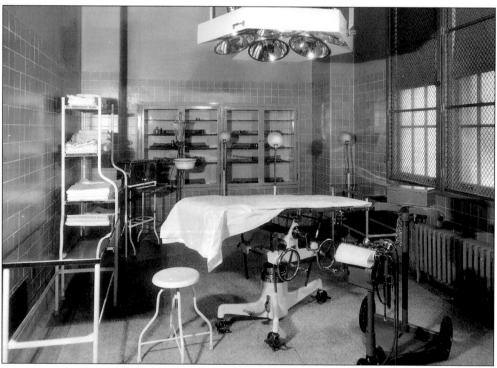

OPERATING ROOM IN "D" BUILDING, 1925. This was state-of-the-art equipment for the time period.

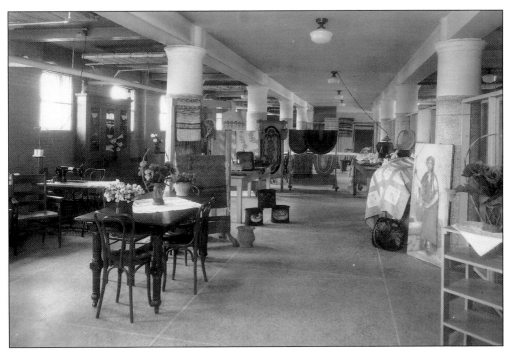

OCCUPATIONAL THERAPY DEPARTMENT, 1929. This department was located in the basement of the Infirmary Building. Rugs and other handicrafts made by patients are displayed.

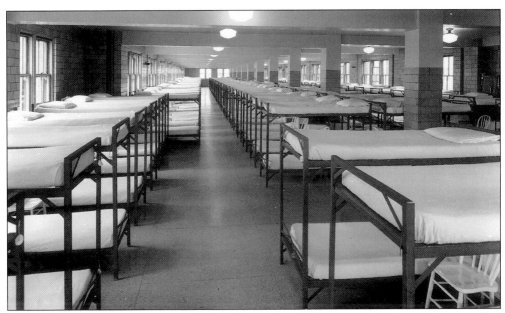

BUNK BEDS IN "N" BUILDING, 1931. Indigents, mainly men, who the employees called *POGIES*—Poor Old Guys in Eloise—were housed in this building. Every winter, the population of these men increased dramatically as they wanted to get in from the cold and get three square meals a day. Those able to work were assigned jobs, such as working in the kitchen, for about four hours a day. Now these people are homeless or living in shelters, a change in social conditions of our times.

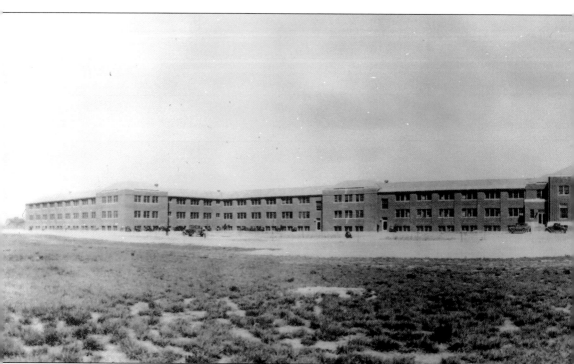

"N" Building or Kelley Hall, the Infirmary Building, 1930s This building was completed in four months in 1930. There were 350 workers on the job daily. This was during the Great Depression when many people were out of work. This huge building was almost 1,000-feet long built in the shape of a double–E. Originally constructed to hold 2,600 people, double wings were added to raise the capacity to over 5,000 people. By November 1931, this

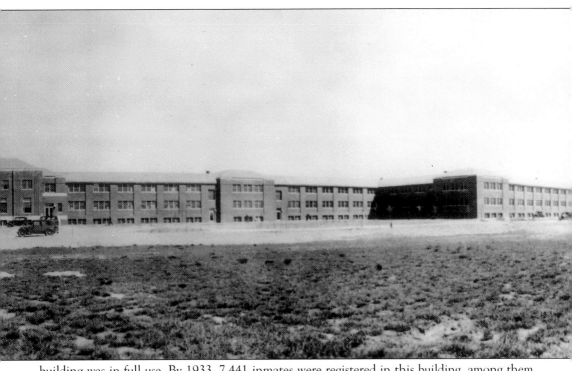

building was in full use. By 1933, 7,441 inmates were registered in this building, among them the blind, crippled or others classified as "infirm," hence the term infirmary. The building even had three jail cells that were used by local police departments. Each jail cell had its own toilet and sink.

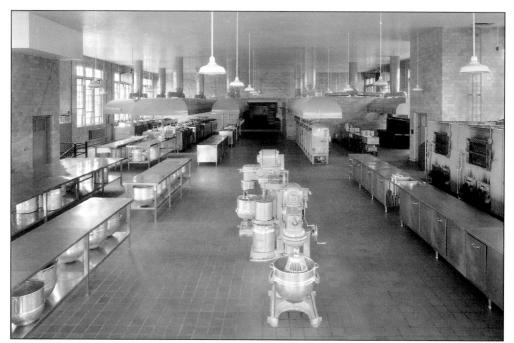

ENLARGED KITCHEN, "N" BUILDING, 1931. The size of the equipment tells it all! The ever-increasing population of the infirmary necessitated doubling the size of the kitchen built in 1930. This kitchen produced thousands of meals a day and was considered the largest institutional kitchen in the United States and probably in the world.

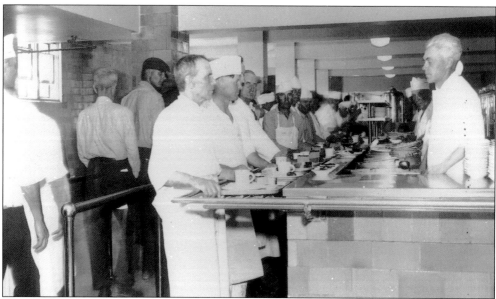

BUDDY, CAN YOU SPARE A HOT LUNCH? Times were hard during the Great Depression and these men are lined up for a meal in the "N" Building cafeteria in 1931. On the menu the day this photo was taken was knackwurst, potato salad with cold boiled eggs, bread, cake, stewed apricots and tea, coffee or milk. They were given as much as they wanted. (Courtesy of the Walter P. Reuther Library, Wayne State University.)

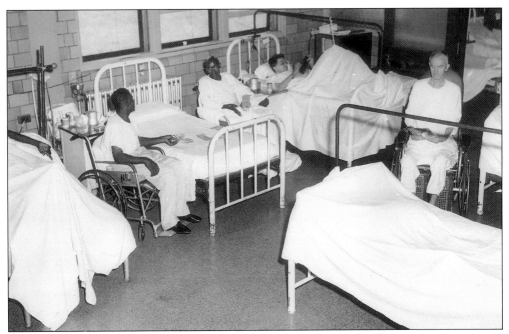

INFIRMARY PATIENTS IN "N" BUILDING, 1950S. These chronically ill patients spent months or even years in Kelley Hall. They passed the time by reading, playing cards, or watching television. Note the early television in the corner.

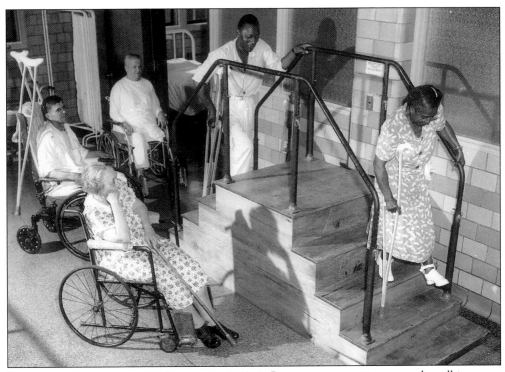

PHYSICAL THERAPY IN "N" BUILDING, 1950S. Patients are practicing crutch walking on a stairway while others wait their turn.

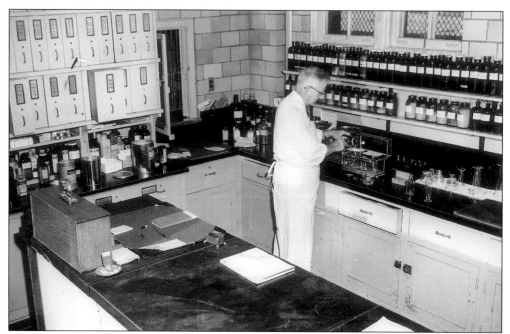

"N" BUILDING PHARMACY, 1952. Pharmacist Mr. Holbert Goldreith is shown dispensing medications in the pharmacy that was located in the basement of "N" Building.

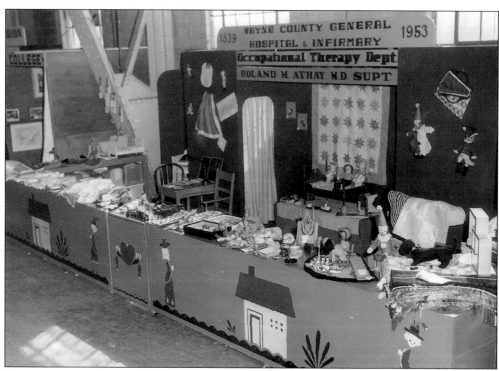

OCCUPATIONAL THERAPY DEPARTMENT, 1953. A display of crafts made by patients is on the tables ready to be sold. The crafts were made as part of the occupational therapy program, which played an important role in the recovery of mental patients.

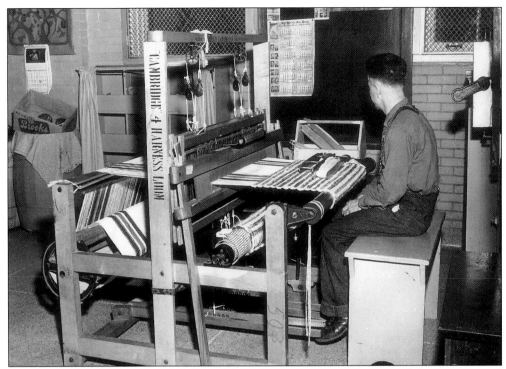

PATIENT AT A LOOM, 1949. This man is making a rug as another part of the occupational therapy program. Every effort was made to encourage patients to engage in activities like this.

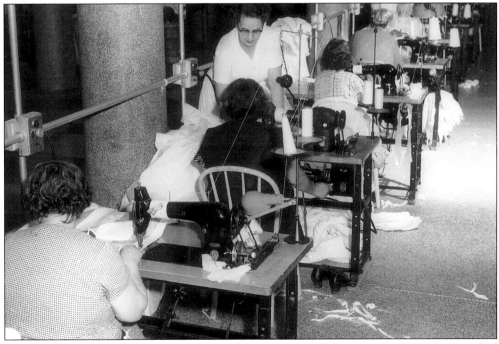

SEWING ROOM, 1952. Sewing was also part of the occupational therapy program. Patients worked on drapes, linens, and bedspreads under the instruction and supervision of Geraldine Eldred.

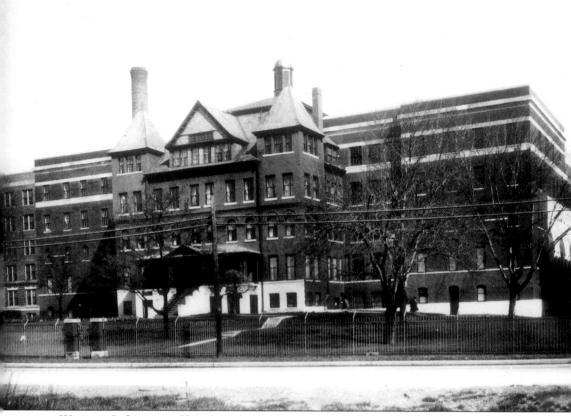

WILLIAM J. SEYMOUR HOSPITAL ("C" BUILDING), 1933. This 534 bed general hospital was established on the site of the Black Horse Tavern and the Fourth County House. The County House was renovated to create this hospital. It was built to service both the patients in the institution who numbered 10,104 at the time, and also to serve the general public in the area. Before this hospital was built, infirmary or mental patients who needed hospitalization had to be taken to the University of Michigan Hospital in Ann Arbor, which was the closest hospital in the area at the time. This hospital even had 50 beds for TB patients. The room rate charged the patients when it opened was $1.13 a day. In the same year, the hospital was approved by the American Medical Association for the training of interns. This was during the Great Depression, so board and laundry were provided to interns, but no salary.

DENTAL UNIT, SEYMOUR HOSPITAL, 1933. Ouch, it hurts just to look at this picture! This was the x-ray room in the new dental clinic. By 1937, there were four full-time dentists who operated two dental clinics at Eloise. Some of the patients worked in these clinics under direct supervision.

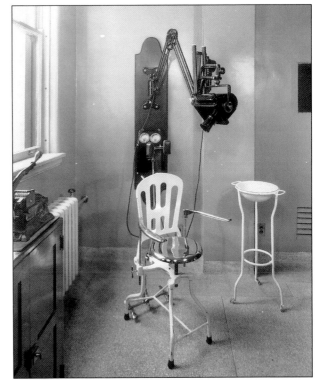

OPERATING ROOM, SEYMOUR HOSPITAL, 1933. This was one of three operating rooms in the new hospital, which boasted all the latest in equipment. Air conditioning was installed in 1934.

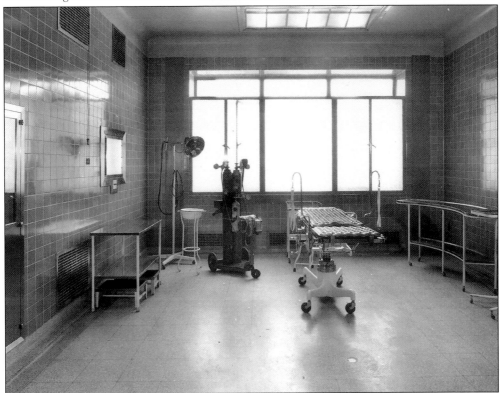

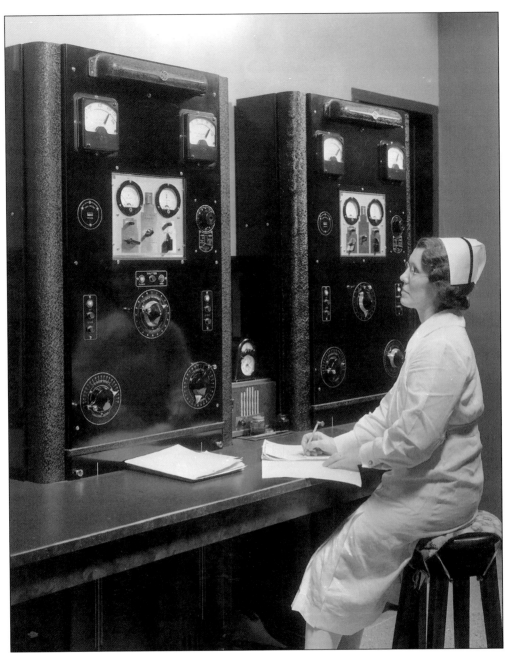

EARLY X-RAY EQUIPMENT AT THE WILLIAM J. SEYMOUR HOSPITAL, 1930S. This is not a scene from a science fiction movie, but it is nurse Mary Gallaher with early x-ray equipment. Eloise was a pioneer in the use of x-rays. W.C. Roentgen, Professor of Physics at the University of Wurzburg in Germany, developed the x-ray (or Roentgen as it as called then) in 1895. Stanislas Keenan was an amateur electrical experimenter and he constructed an x-ray machine in December 1896, which was used in the County House dispensary. Members of the Wayne County Medical Society visited the institution and Detroit-area physicians sent patients to the hospital for x-rays of fractures. Eloise was among the first, if not the first, medical facility in the U.S. to use x-rays for diagnosis.

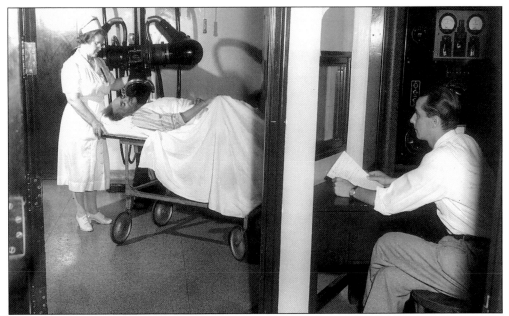

X-Ray Department, Seymour Hospital, 1952. Nurse Mary Gallaher positions the patient for a deep therapy treatment. Deep therapy was a form of radiation used to treat cancer. Dr. Joseph Zbikowski, a radiologist, is in the x-ray booth.

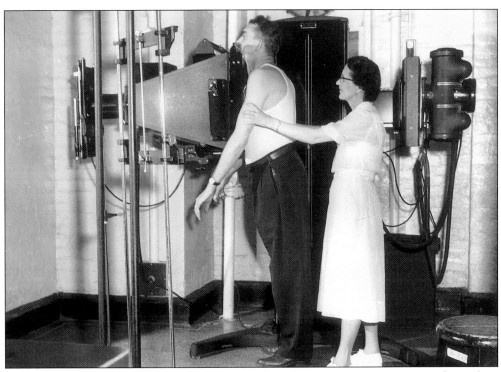

Patient Receiving a Chest X-Ray, 1952. A technician positions a patient for a chest x-ray. This was the state of the art equipment in 1952. This department gave 17,917 x-ray examinations to patients in 1952.

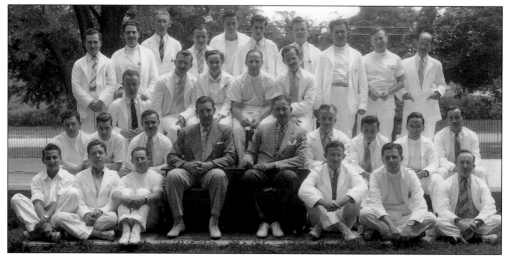

ELOISE HOSPITAL STAFF, 1939. Posed on the front lawn of the hospital are members of the medical staff. Drs. C.L.R. Pearman and Robert Jennings are in the front row wearing suits. In the third row, far left, is Dr. Eugene Quigley. In the last row, far right, is Dr. Bogucz.

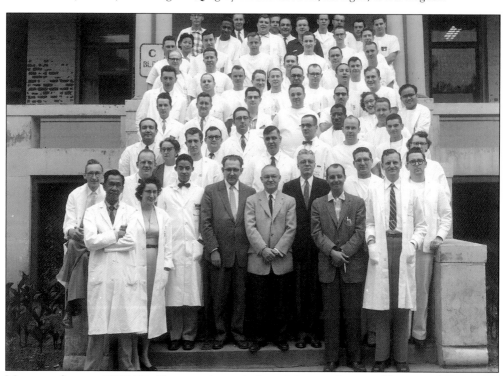

MEDICAL STAFF, 1956-57. Doctors pictured, from left to right, are: (front row) Primativo Rivera, John A. Belisle, Sylvester E. Gould, Douglas B. McDowell, Joseph Zbikowski and Julius Kaupas; (second row) W.N. Davis, Wayne "Will" Glas, and E. J. Conklin; (third row) Morteza Minui, Natalia Janicki, Harold Oster, Merlin Townley, Pierre Martel, and Norman Nelson; (fourth row) Stanley Olejniczak (second) and Vladimir Kozlowski; (fifth row, third from left) George Mertz; (second from top row) Yoeh Ming Ting, and Bela Szappanyos; (top row center) Victor M. Azuela.

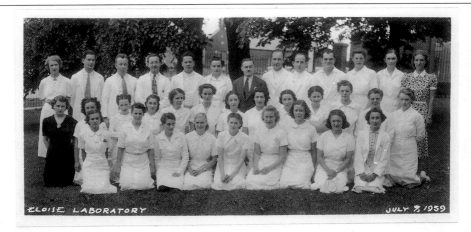

TOP ROW: F.VERNOR DR.M.DALE DR.E.QUIGLEY DR.H.A.SHECKET DR. R. KUHN
DR.S.E.GOULD DR.D.SILER DR.SIMONS G.LANE M.HUFF H.CHURCH E.SCHWARZ
MIDDLE ROW: M.CHERNAK M. BERNSTEIN M. KERCHER H. ROSEN
G. KERCHER A. DEARNLEY J. MILLER L.FURMAN M. REEDER
M. TRESE D. PAULSON T. ABBENSETH E. FREEBORN
LOWER ROW: H. PELOK M. KLEIN R. SENESAC J. COONRATH
F. PEARCE P. GUIDER M. CALL L. RUPP M. LINDENBAUM

GROUP PHOTOS OF LABORATORY PERSONNEL. These two group photos show the laboratory staff in 1939 and 1960. Staff shown in the photo dated June 8, 1960 are, from left to right, top row and down: Theresa O'Leary, Grace Kercher, Shirley Dye, Frank Sartin, Barbara Keen, Judith Murphy, Alice Miller, Rhea Schroeder, Doris Miller, Felix Malotha, Percy Fuller, Shirley Crump, Robert Mohr, Lynett Tracy, James Hill, Ann Ruffer, Patricia Steward, Henry Higgins, Dorothy Grahek, Joyce Julian, Leonard Johnson, Mary Jones, Ann Copeland, Louis Kovach, Barbara Lanning, Patricia Rice, Carmen Charpentier, Winifred Byrd, Frances Gaines, Elizabeth Reed, Lynn Baril, Jesse F. Goodwin, Ph.D., Frank Ellis, M.D., S.E. Gould, M.D., Irene Block, and Myrtle Buckley.

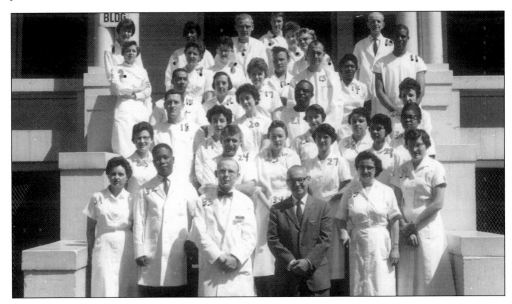

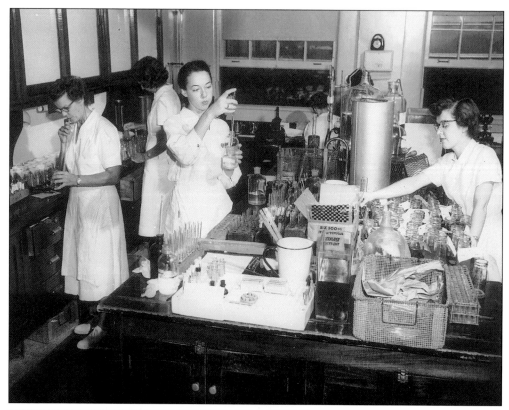

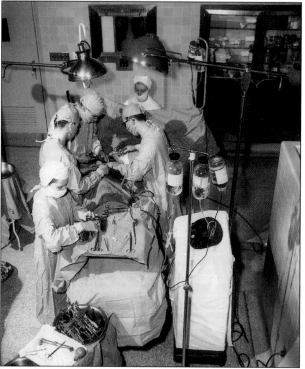

MEDICAL DIAGNOSTIC LABORATORY, 1952. Laboratory employees are performing testing. The hospital laboratories also did the testing for the Wayne County Health Department.

THE OPERATING ROOM AT THE WILLIAM J. SEYMOUR HOSPITAL, 1952. The patient is having surgery for chest cancer. This hospital performed 4,000 major operations and 2,000 minor operations in 1952. Dr. Merle Musselman was the Director of Emergency Surgery.

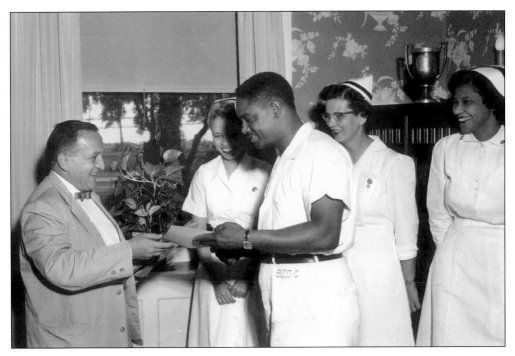

Dr. Samuel D. Jacobson Presenting Awards to Hospital Staff, 1950s. Dr. Jacobson was the General Superintendent of Eloise, later known as Wayne County General Hospital and the Walter P. Reuther Memorial Long Term Care Facility, from October 22, 1953 to May 24, 1965. He married Miss Delores Gallagher, R.N., the nursing supervisor of the outpatient clinics, after a long courtship. The presentation and the party that followed were held in the superintendent's home, which was on the grounds.

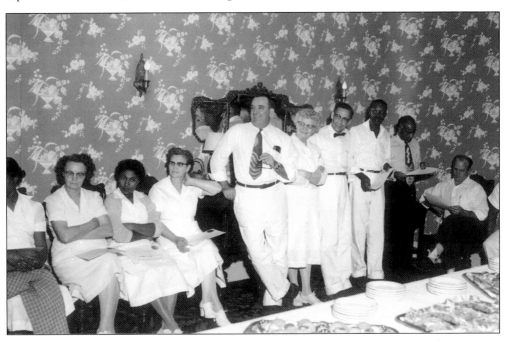

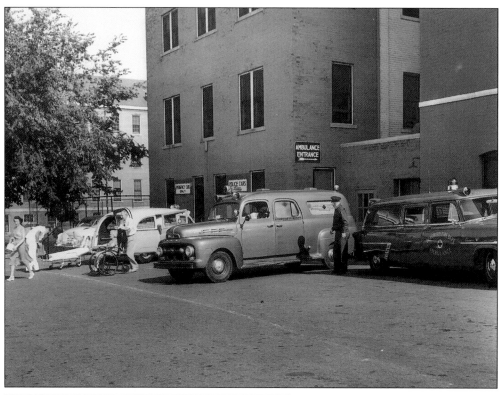

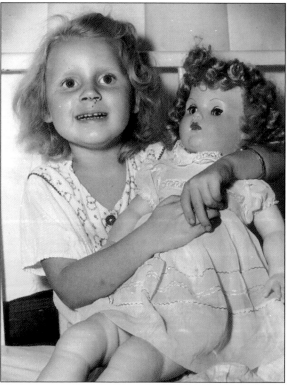

AMBULANCE ENTRANCE, SEYMOUR HOSPITAL, 1952. The Emergency Room and Admitting were in "B" Building, which adjoined the Seymour Hospital, or "C" Building. Three ambulances, one from the Dearborn Fire Department, attest to just how busy this hospital was.

A LITTLE PATIENT, 1952. This unidentified little girl holding her doll was a patient at the William J. Seymour Hospital. Both the Seymour Hospital and later the Wayne County General Hospital had pediatric units. The Seymour Hospital's pediatric unit was located in "B" Building along with admitting and the emergency room.

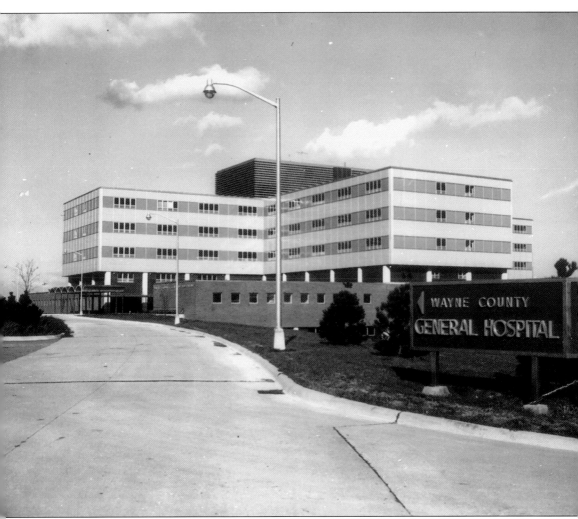

WAYNE COUNTY GENERAL HOSPITAL AND HEALTH CENTER ("O" BUILDING), 1962. This 500-bed acute care hospital, which was located on Merriman Road, opened in 1962 and served as the major trauma hospital for western Wayne County until its closure in 1984. It cost $15 million to build. It was affiliated with Wayne State University and then the University of Michigan. There were 11 operating rooms and 10 x-ray units. It also housed the first kidney dialysis unit in the State of Michigan. It was the second hospital in Michigan to do a kidney transplant in 1964. Its doors were opened to all and no one was ever turned away for lack of insurance or funds. The hospital was connected to the Wayne County Health Department. Both buildings were razed in 2000.

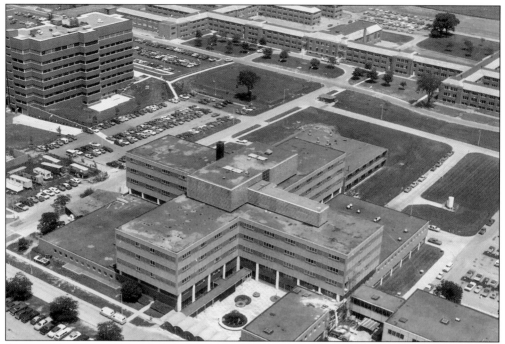

AERIAL VIEW OF WAYNE COUNTY GENERAL HOSPITAL, C. 1974. Wayne County General Hospital and Health Center is seen in the foreground, with the new Walter P. Reuther Memorial Long Term Care facility to the left and "N" Building (or the old Infirmary Building) in the background.

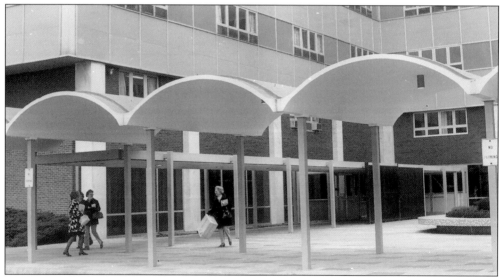

MAIN ENTRANCE TO WAYNE COUNTY GENERAL HOSPITAL, 1962. The six-floor hospital had 350,000 square feet of space. The first two floors were brick and marble and the top three floors were enameled steel in two shades of green. The outpatient clinics, adult and pediatric, were housed to the left on the first floor of the building. The emergency room, admitting, x-ray, the laboratories, dental clinic, administrative offices, chapel, physical therapy, occupational therapy, credit, social services, and gift shop were all housed on the first floor.

MAIN LOBBY OF WAYNE COUNTY GENERAL HOSPITAL, 1962. The curved wall with blue mosaic tile was the focal point of the lobby and waiting room area. (Courtesy of the Walter P. Reuther Library, Wayne State University.)

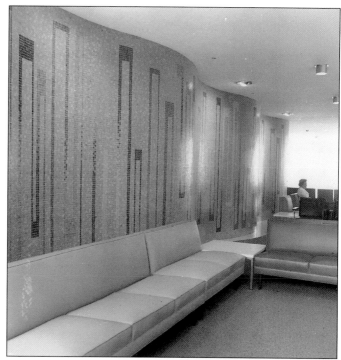

PATIENT WARD, WAYNE COUNTY GENERAL HOSPITAL, 1962. Elizabeth A. Finnigan, Director of Nurses, and Gloria Cotton, R.N., inspect a four-bed ward in the new hospital. The patient rooms contained one to five beds, though most were four bed wards. (Courtesy of the Walter P. Reuther Library, Wayne State University.)

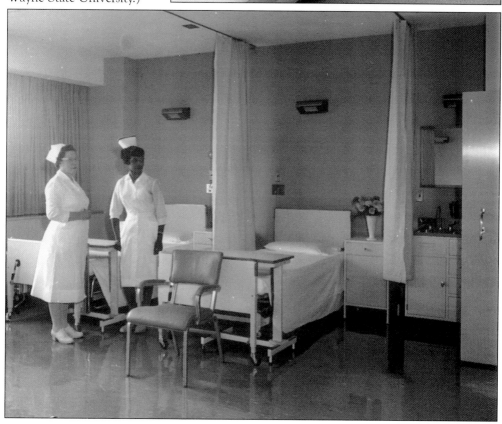

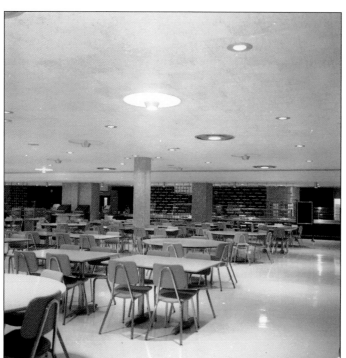

CAFETERIA, WAYNE COUNTY GENERAL HOSPITAL, 1962. Employees and visitors used this cafeteria. It was a busy and crowded place most days of the week. Private dining rooms were used for staff meetings and parties. (Courtesy of the Walter P. Reuther Library, Wayne State University.)

PEDIATRIC UNIT, WAYNE COUNTY GENERAL HOSPITAL, 1960s. A nurse and attendant care for young patients in the general hospital's pediatric unit. There was also a pediatric emergency room and outpatient clinic that serviced the western Wayne County area.

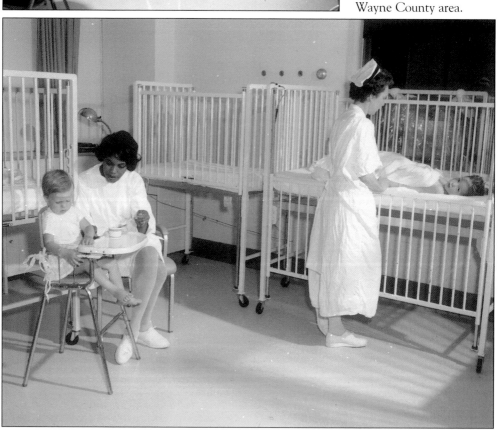

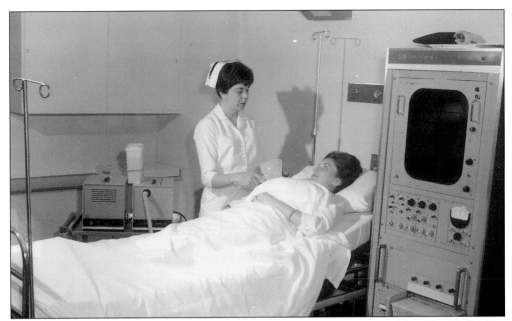

INTENSIVE CARE UNIT, WAYNE COUNTY GENERAL HOSPITAL, 1960s. Nurse Pat Gallagher, R.N. monitors an intensive care patient with what was then the latest in high-tech equipment. The hospital had both an intensive care and a cardiac care unit, which were located on the second floor of the hospital.

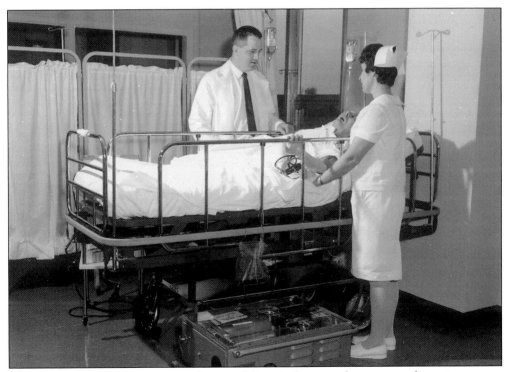

RESPIRATOR PATIENT, INTENSIVE CARE, 1960s. A doctor and nurse attend a patient on an early respirator. The respirator is the box on the floor.

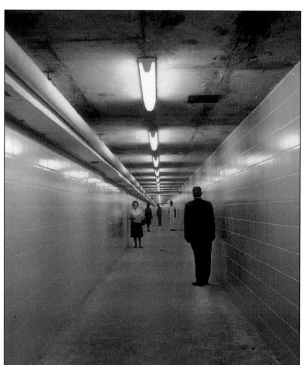

Tunnel Connecting the General Hospital with Other Buildings, 1962. This 800-foot tunnel connected the General Hospital with "N" Building and later the Walter P. Reuther Long Term Care Facility. It was used for employees and for patient transport between buildings. (Courtesy of the Walter P. Reuther Library, Wayne State University.)

Walter P. Reuther Long Tern Care Facility ("P" Building), 1974. This 350-bed facility replaced the Infirmary ("N" Building) for housing the chronically ill. There were six patient floors. This building was taken over by the State of Michigan in 1980 to care for chronically ill psychiatric patients and it is still used for this purpose.

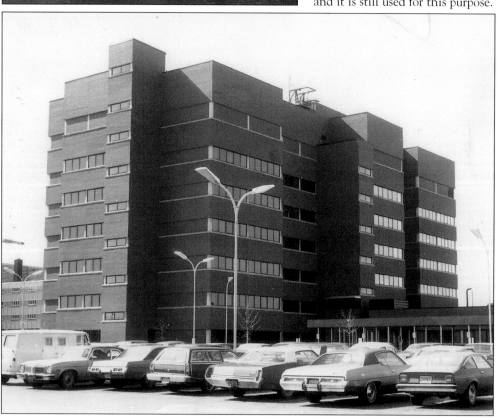

Four

A City in Itself

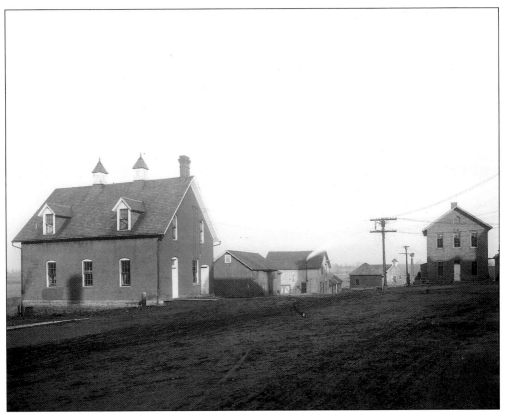

VIEW OF THE GROUNDS, 1912. Eloise appears as the little village it was in this photo of some miscellaneous buildings on the grounds. Shown, from left to right, are the old carpenter shop, the hard coal house, the first sewage disposal plant, the round house (morgue), the pigpen, and the schoolhouse.

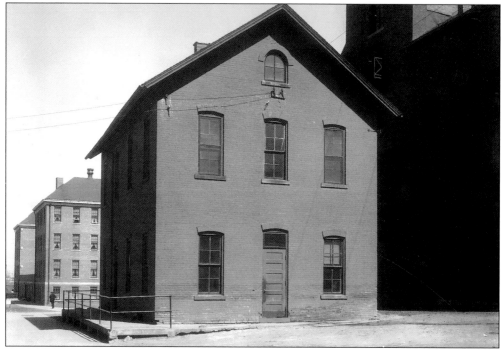

SCHOOLHOUSE, 1880–1887. Young children whose parents had died of cholera were among the first inmates. Teaching these students *reading, writing and ciphering* was one of the duties of the seamstress. There was an unofficial school in a designated area from 1839 to 1861. Officially designated as School District #10 in Nankin Township in 1861, by 1898 school age children were no longer accepted and the school was closed.

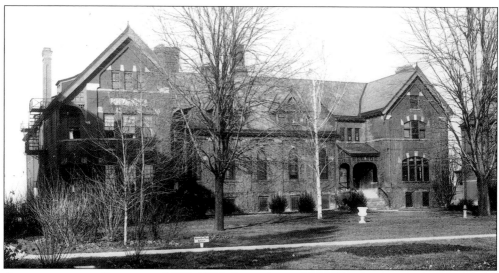

ADMINISTRATION BUILDING, 1887–1888. It was located between the County House and the Asylum Building. The first floor contained offices, and the west wing was used for open wards for the male insane. The post office was located in the east wing. A chapel was in the center of the building. There was a storeroom and butcher shop in the basement. The building was razed in 1930 and "D" Building was put up almost exactly in the same place in 1931.

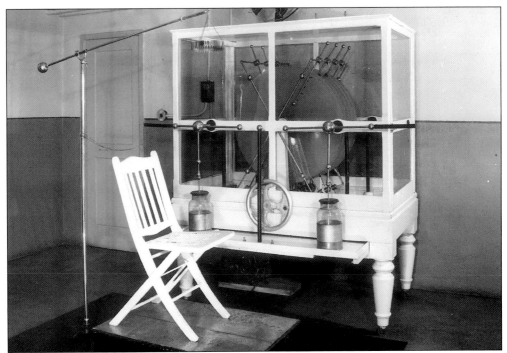

REASSEMBLED ELECTRICAL LABORATORY, 1921. The sector-less Wimhurst machine that was designed by Stanislas M. Keenan in 1896-7 is shown as reassembled. It was originally housed in the rear of the County House dispensary. Keenan carried out the first early experiments with the roentgen ray or x-ray and at the time of his death had an extensive collection from the old Crookes tubes to the latest in x-ray equipment.

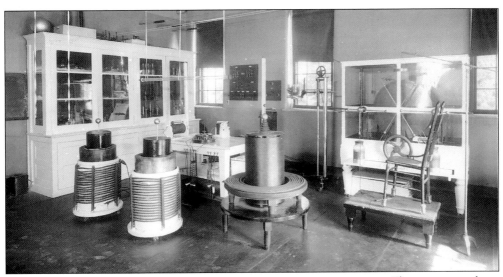

SECTIONAL VIEW OF THE REMODELED TRANSFORMER ROOM, 1921. The superintendents would bring friends from Detroit to see this room. Unsuspecting visitors who were seated in an innocent looking chair would be given a jolt of electricity much to the amusement of the superintendents who were in on the joke. Many high school classes were also taken here to gain knowledge of electricity.

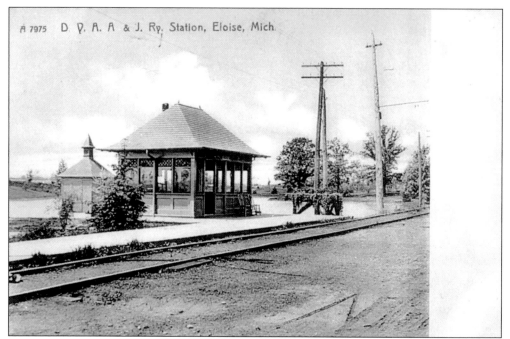

A 7975   D. Y. A. A. & J. Ry. Station, Eloise, Mich.

THE DETROIT-YPSILANTI AND ANN ARBOR RAILROAD STATION, EARLY 1900S. The Detroit-Ypsilanti and Ann Arbor Railroad had a line of electric cars that reached as far as Ann Arbor. The first cars reached Eloise in 1898, enabling better access for visitors from Detroit. This is the Interurban Station for Eloise on a penny postcard printed by the Rotograph Company of New York City.

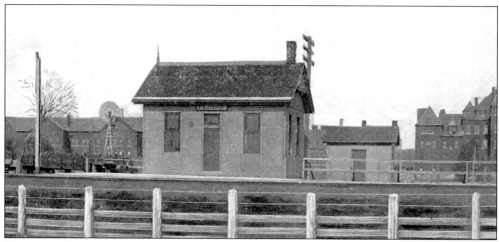

MICHIGAN CENTRAL RAILWAY DEPOT, 1895. The station was built in 1886. The last passenger car ran through Eloise in 1929. Freight cars continued to go through for some time afterwards. In the background, the Asylum is on the left, and the County House is on the right.

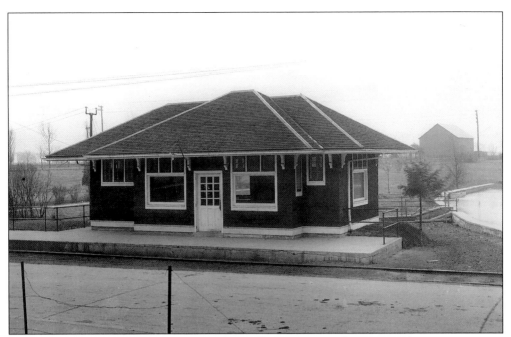

Eloise Trolley Station, c. 1930. The trolley was a popular means of transportation at a time when most people did not own automobiles. The trolley station was built in 1911. It contained two toilet rooms, a storeroom, cigar and confectionery stand, and a public telephone station. In the background is a frame barn that was built in 1875, and at the time the trolley station was built, was the oldest building at Eloise.

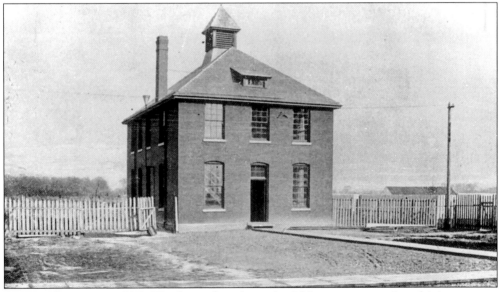

Asylum Laundry, 1895. The lower floor housed a 20-horsepower engine, driving a steam mangle, a centrifugal extractor and three washing machines. The second floor had a steam dryer and a general ironing outfit. It was used until 1910 when the County House Power Laundry was built. This building then became the Fire Hall in 1930 and it is the oldest building still standing on the grounds.

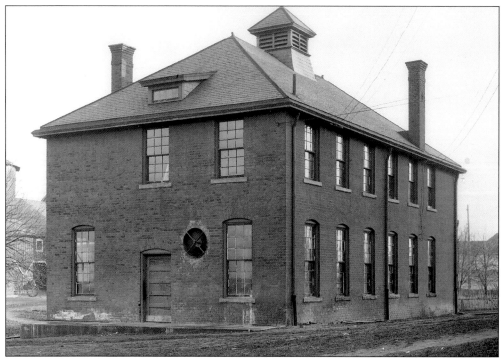

COUNTY HOUSE POWER LAUNDRY, 1896. This was the laundry for the County House until 1910 and then it merged with the Asylum laundry. It was converted into inmates' quarters in 1917 and was torn down in 1931.

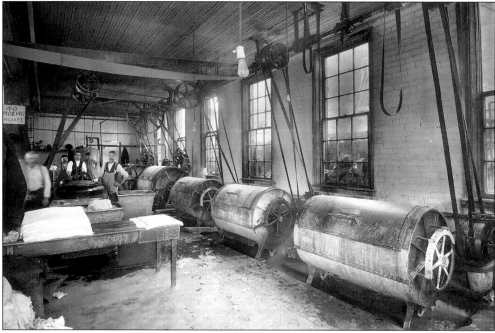

INTERIOR OF LAUNDRY, 1913. These men are laundering sheets. The cylindrical containers are the mammoth washers.

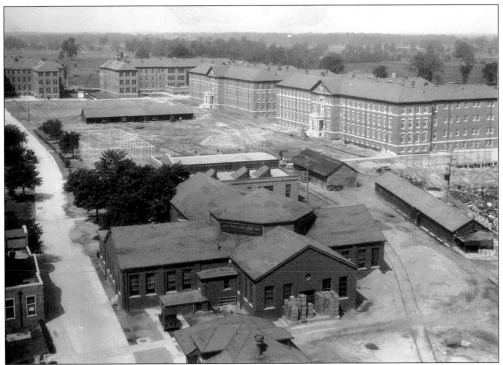

New Laundry, 1930. At the time this laundry was erected in 1916, there were 55 buildings at Eloise and the old laundry had reached and passed its capacity. The building was in the form of a cross with the major axis east and west. It was built in an orchard to the rear of Hospital Building "B." In the background to the right are "L" and "M" Buildings. It was later called the Trades Building.

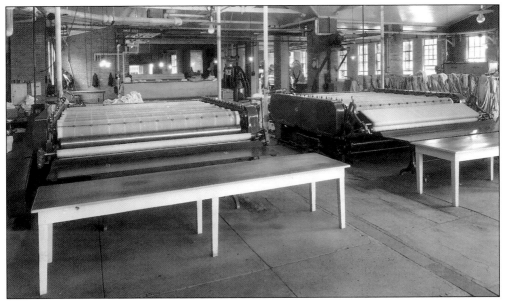

Interior of New Laundry, 1930. Eight-roll flat work ironers are shown in the new laundry. With 55 buildings on the grounds, there were plenty of sheets that needed ironing.

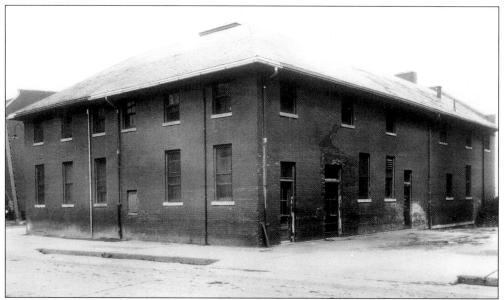

THE BAKERY, BUILT 1905. The first baking at the County House was done in a mud oven in 1841. This bakery, one of few buildings still standing, had additions put on in 1917 and 1931. It had a steam room for raising bread. In 1931, a doughnut-making machine was added. The bakery closed in 1960 and the hospital began purchasing baked goods from outside vendors.

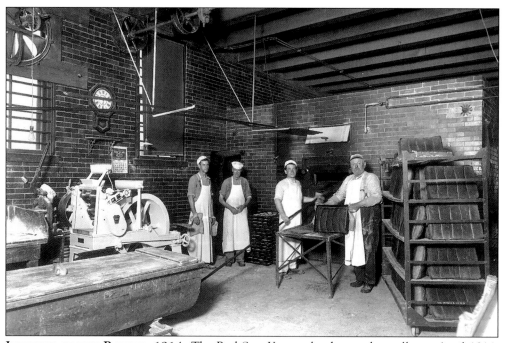

INTERIOR OF THE BAKERY, 1914. The Red Star Yeast calendar on the wall says April 1914. Many people had fond memories of the aroma of the newly baked bread emanating from the open door. To the far right is Walter Prosser, who was the bakery supervisor. In 1912, this bakery produced, among other things, 154,502 loaves of bread, two pounds to the loaf; 10,187 dozen buns; 27,874 pounds of ginger cake; 21,318 dozen cookies and 9,303 pies.

THE POWER PLANT, 1912. The first smokestack, 50-feet high, was built in 1894 and the chimney was raised 30 feet three years later. The powerhouse provided steam heating to all the buildings on the complex. The steam it provided through underground tunnels circulated through all the radiators in the buildings.

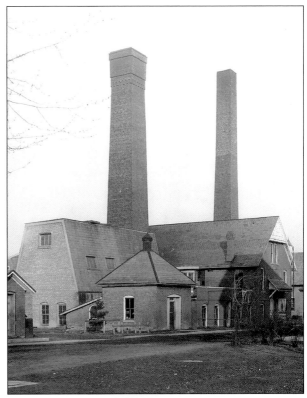

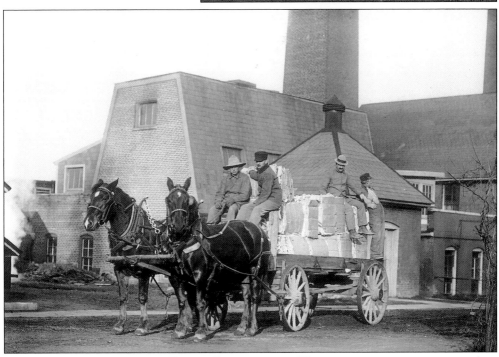

WORKMEN IN FRONT OF THE POWER PLANT, 1912. These teamsters, seen posing in their wagon in front of the power plant, are hauling a load of supplies.

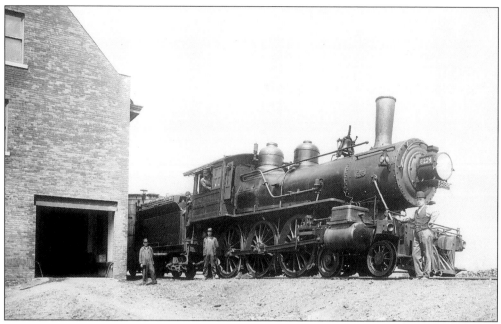

MICHIGAN CENTRAL FREIGHT TRAIN, 1913. Railroad workers stand with a train on the trestle that was constructed in 1912-13. The train delivered coal to the powerhouse.

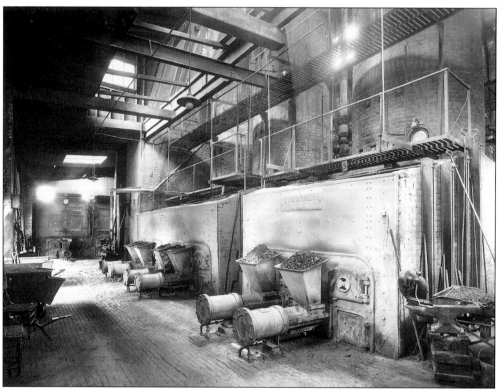

BOILER ROOM AND STOKER, 1921. These boilers were fed by coal brought in by the Michigan Central Railroad that had a sidetrack to the rear of the boiler house.

NEW POWERHOUSE, 1923. It was built entirely around the old power plant, which was gradually dismantled as work progressed. A new smokestack was constructed that was 200-feet high. This smokestack and powerhouse still exists. The powerhouse made history in 1924, when it became one of the first hospital-based generators in the United States. It supplied all the light, heat, power and hot water for the institution.

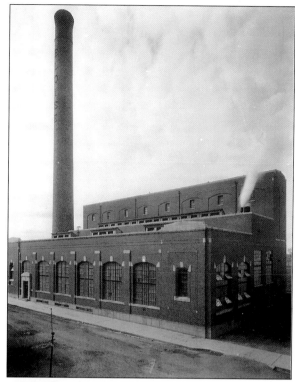

DYNAMO ROOM, 1924. In contrast to the boiler room in the old power plant, this room was so clean one could eat off the floor.

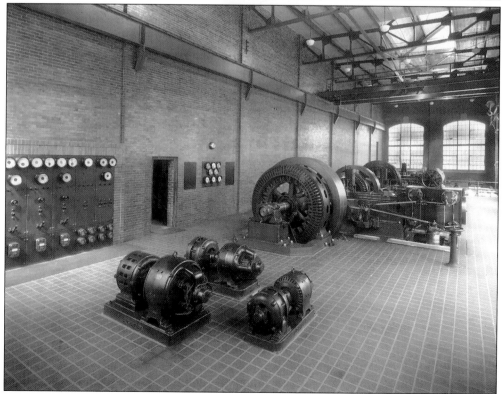

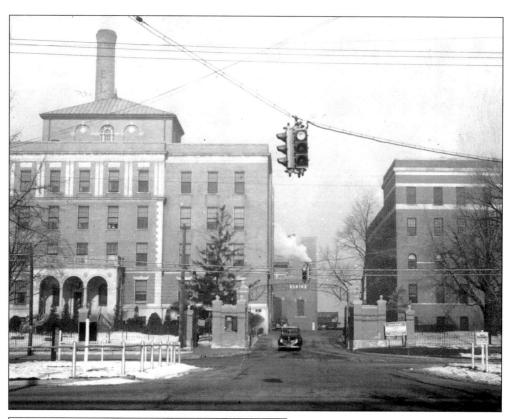

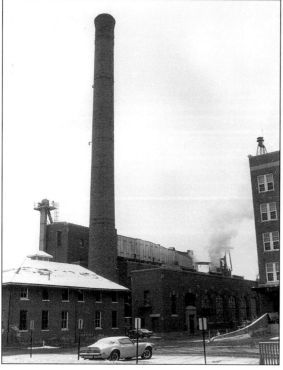

VIEW OF POWER PLANT AT ENTRANCE TO ELOISE, 1940S. To the left is "D" Building and to the right is the William J. Seymour Hospital ("C" Building.) The power plant can be seen in the center of the photo beyond the gate with the smokestack behind "D" Building.

VIEW OF POWER PLANT, 1970S. A light coating of snow covers the cars on this wintry day adding atmosphere to this photograph. The bakery is to the left and the power plant and smokestack are to the right. Part of "D" Building can also be seen on the far right.

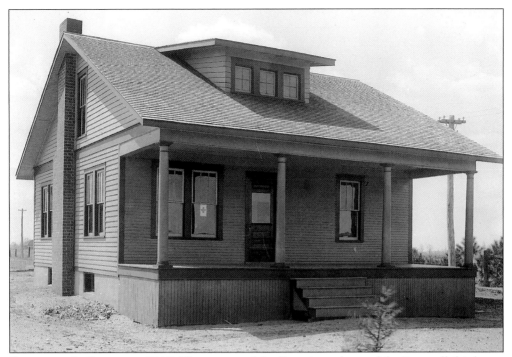

SWINEHERD'S COTTAGE, 1918. The reports of the Superintendents of the Poor call this house the Swineherd's Cottage. Other records refer to it as the Gardener's Cottage. Either way, it was used to house farm employees and was located south of the Michigan Central tracks near the frame barn.

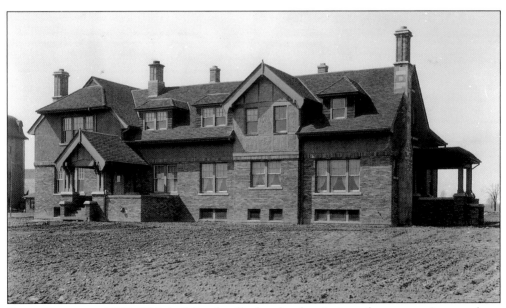

FARM COTTAGE, 1926. This building hardly fits the description of a cottage. It was a large duplex. Bert Randall, the farm manager lived on one side and George Rogers, who managed the diary herd, lived on the other side. The second floor was a dormitory for farm hands that paid $26-a-month room and board. It was later used for general employee housing.

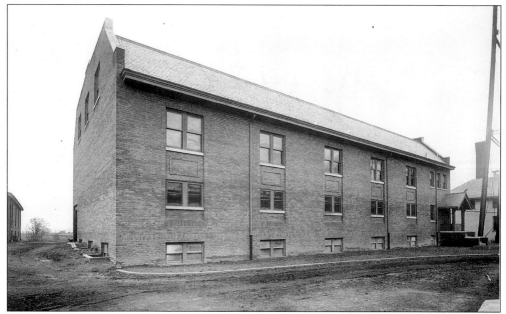

AMUSEMENT HALL AND STOREROOM, 1912. This building contained a basement, a storeroom on the first floor, and an amusement hall on the second floor. Part of the basement was used for storage and a large butcher shop, and part contained a bowling alley. The bowling alley and a movie theater both opened in 1914 providing entertainment for employees and patients. Dances were also held here every two weeks.

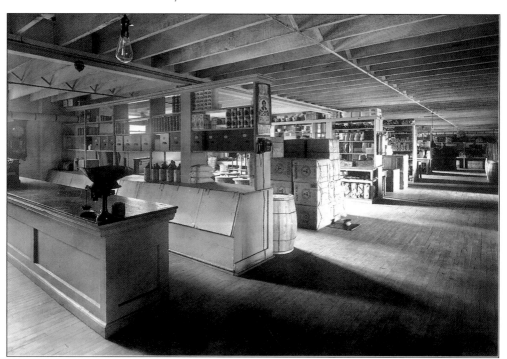

INTERIOR OF THE GENERAL STORE, C. 1913. The general store provided everything needed by all the buildings on the Eloise grounds.

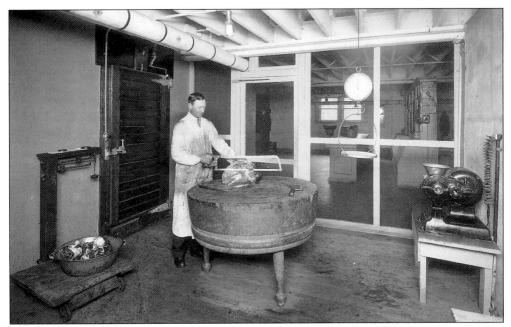

MEAT ROOM IN THE GENERAL STORE, C. 1913. A butcher is carving some meat to be used in one of the many kitchens on the grounds.

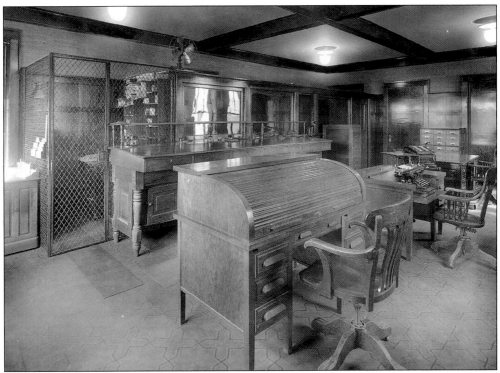

GENERAL OFFICE, 1917. This is a view of the general office that was located in the Administration Building. It was expanded and renovated in 1917 and oak paneling was put up and new linoleum was laid on the floors.

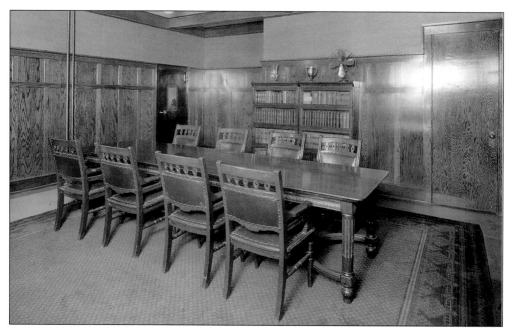

BOARD ROOM IN THE ADMINISTRATION BUILDING, 1917. Here is where the governing board of the institution met. Oak paneling was put up and new linoleum was laid in 1917. The interior rooms of many of the Eloise buildings were crafted of fine woods and were nicely appointed.

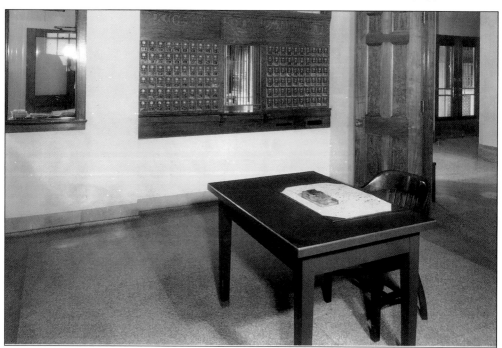

POST OFFICE, 1931. The post office was first established in 1894 and was in the Administration Building before moving to "D" Building in 1931. Mail sent from here was postmarked *Eloise*. The zip code was 48132. The post office closed in 1979 when there was a drop in mail volume due to fewer patients and employees. After that, mail was handled by the Westland Post Office.

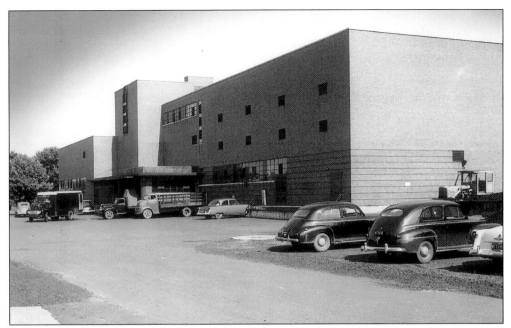

THE NEW WAREHOUSE. This building was built in 1936 and was more commonly called the Commissary. It served as the focal point for the delivery and distribution of all equipment and supplies to the institution. This building is currently being used as a homeless shelter.

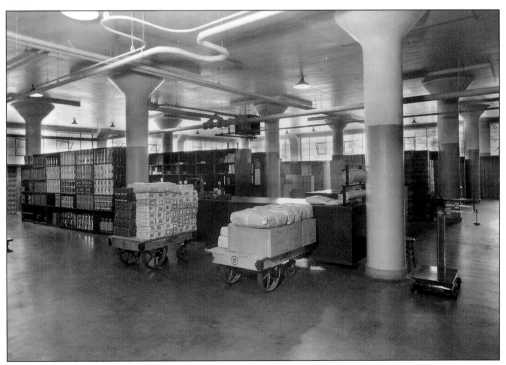

GROCERY DISTRIBUTING ROOM, 1936. This room was in the Commissary or New Warehouse building. Groceries were provided from here to all the kitchens in the buildings. Every building housing patients had its own kitchen.

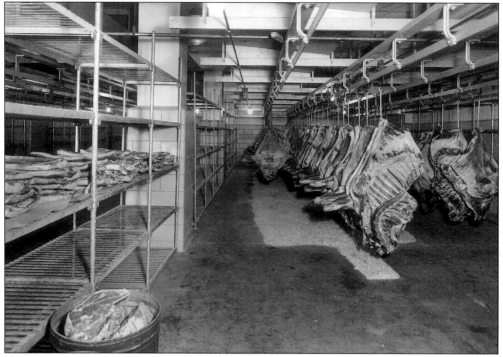

COLD STORAGE MEAT ROOM, 1936. This is another room in the Commissary, where large supplies of meat were kept on hand to feed all the employees and patients at Eloise.

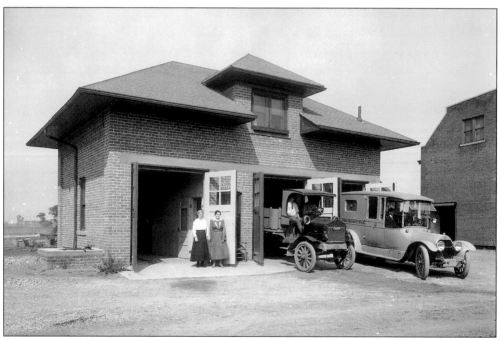

AMBULANCE GARAGE, 1918. Two ladies pose for the camera in front of the building. The *Eloise Hospital* Cadillac ambulance was stored here. The ambulance cost $3,500. The second floor contained a suite of three rooms. Part of the Amusement Hall can be seen at the right.

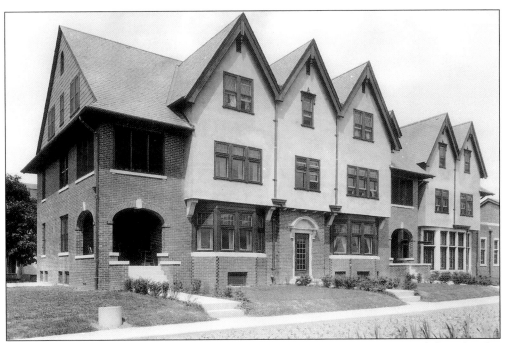

APARTMENT BUILDING AND CAFETERIA, 1921. Built in the Domestic English style, this three-story brick and stucco building contained living quarters for four families and double rooms for unmarried help. The cafeteria was on the first floor at the north end of the building. Most of the employees took their meals in the cafeteria.

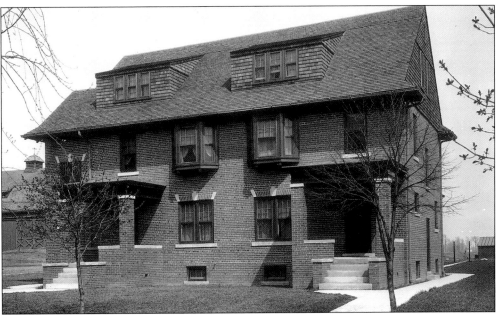

TERRACE BUILDING, 1923. This is a view to the south of the first addition to the Terrace Building. There were two family apartments, and the attic story contained five bedrooms for employees, bath and toilet rooms. The family apartments contained three bedrooms. About 20 percent of the employees lived on the grounds. Many employees also resided in the surrounding communities.

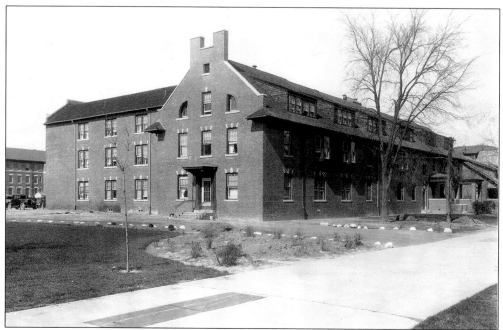

NEW TERRACE BUILDING, 1928. This view shows the addition put on in 1928. Each of the three floors contained 11 double and one single room, together with toilet, wash, linen, tub, trunk, and utility rooms.

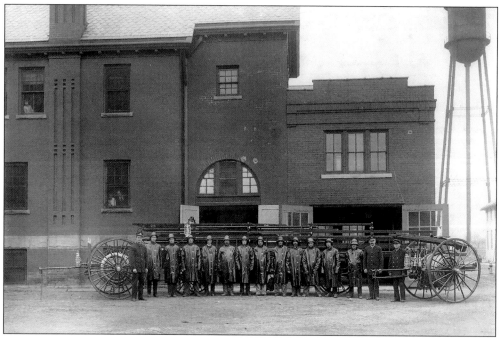

ELOISE FIRE DEPARTMENT, 1912. The Eloise Fire Department was officially founded in 1909 under the direction of a professional fireman. The fire chief was John Gilmore, second to the right, who had been a member of the Detroit Fire Department. On the far left is Assistant Chief Merrell. They were all wearing new oilskin coats and hats. Note the water tower in the background.

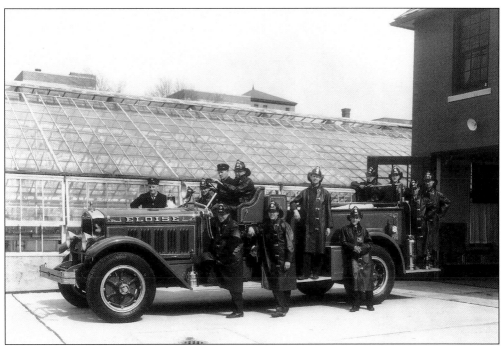

ELOISE FIRE DEPARTMENT, 1933. This photo, taken in 1932, shows the new $12,500 American LaFrance truck with a V-12 cylinder, 121-horsepower engine. At the same time other equipment, such as firemen's clothing, was purchased. Up to 1978 the fire department consisted of 18 men, the same number as the first fire brigade in 1898. Don Dickerson is third from left on the running board. One of the Eloise greenhouses is in the background.

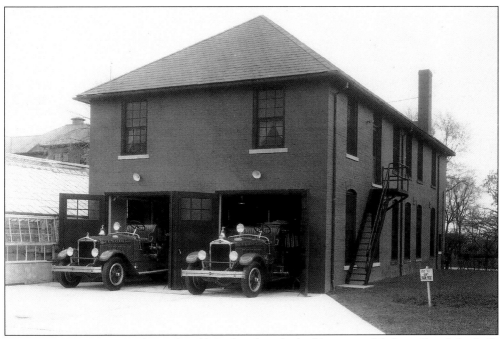

NEW FIRE HALL, 1933. This is the old Asylum laundry building remodeled as a "new" fire hall.

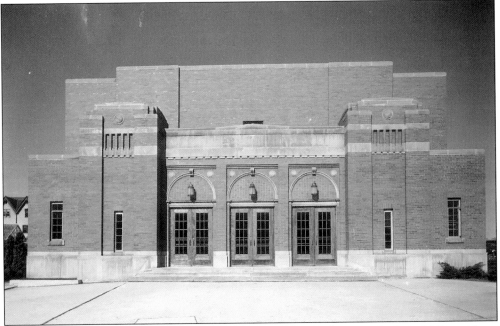

THE T.K. GRUBER MEMORIAL AUDITORIUM, 1940. The Auditorium, built in 1940 and later named for Dr. Gruber, was used for patient and employee performances, such as ballet and dance recitals, fashion shows, and church services. Concerts by a Dr. X, a patient in the music therapy program, were broadcast from the Gruber Auditorium over two radio stations on a nationwide transmission.

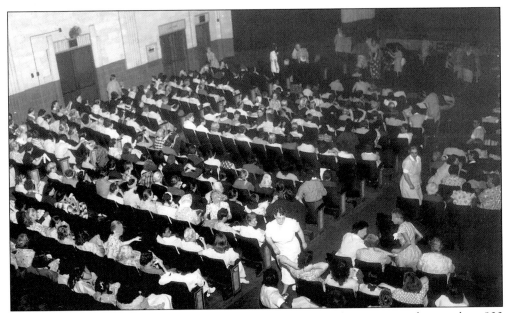

FULL HOUSE IN THE GRUBER AUDITORIUM, 1940S. The auditorium seated more than 900 people. Here a group of female patients are attending one of the bi-weekly movie showings. Big name performers also put on shows for the Eloise patients when they were in Detroit appearing at the Fox Theater.

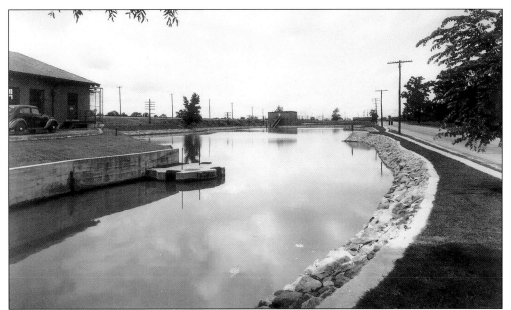

FIRST ARTIFICIAL LAKE. A source of water was needed for Eloise, and in 1893 a dam was built to create this lake. A Catholic cemetery had been located where the lake was formed and the remains were moved. The lake was also used to make ice, and one of the icehouses can be seen at the top of the lake. The building is the water softening plant, which was built in 1924. Michigan Avenue is the road on the right.

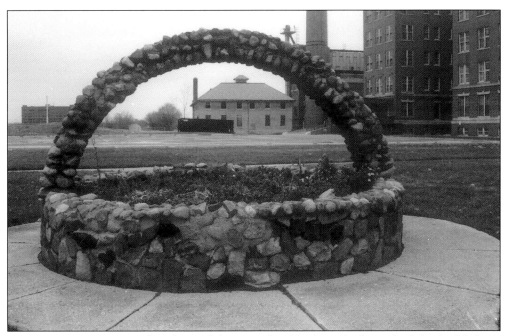

STONE FLORAL BASKET. This photo of the stone floral basket, which was built by the Hudsons to display flowers, frames the old bakery in the background. "D" Building is shown to the right and part of the smokestack and powerhouse can be seen in the background. The Walter P. Reuther Memorial Long Term Care Facility is in the distance.

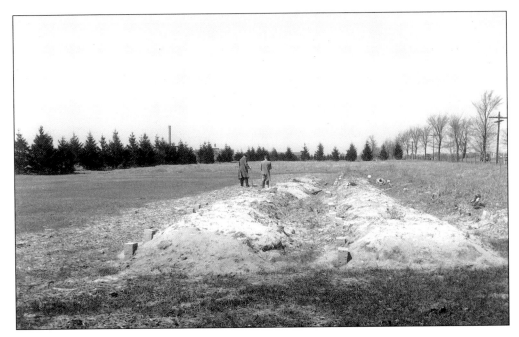

ELOISE CEMETERY, 1948. About 7,100 people were buried in the Eloise Cemetery between 1910 and 1948. These were patients who died at the institution and had no known relatives and/or relatives who were unwilling or unable to bury them. Only numbered blocks identify the graves. After 1948, all unclaimed bodies were sent to the Wayne State University College of Medicine and no further burials were made there. (Courtesy of the Walter P. Reuther Library, Wayne State University.)

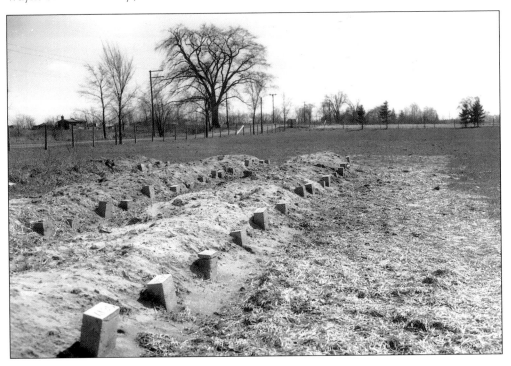

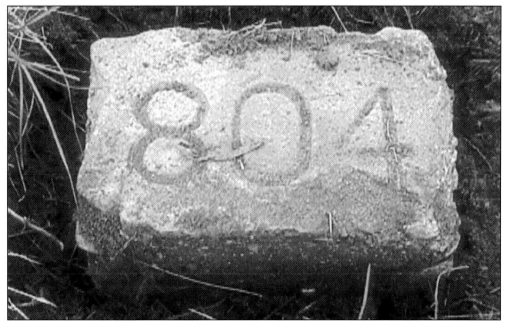

GRAVE MARKER 804, ELOISE CEMETERY. No one knows who is buried in this grave. Most of the records of those buried here were lost or misplaced.

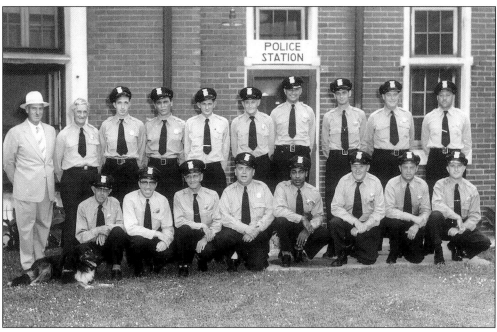

ELOISE POLICE DEPARTMENT, 1952. Mr. Louis O'Brien, in civilian clothes at far left, a retired inspector from the Detroit Police Department, was employed as a Detective Lieutenant and he developed the institutional guard force into a professional-appearing and trained body. He had periodic group photos taken. Bill Anderson is at the far right in the second row. Missing from this photo is William Hancock. Both of these men later became chief of the hospital security department.

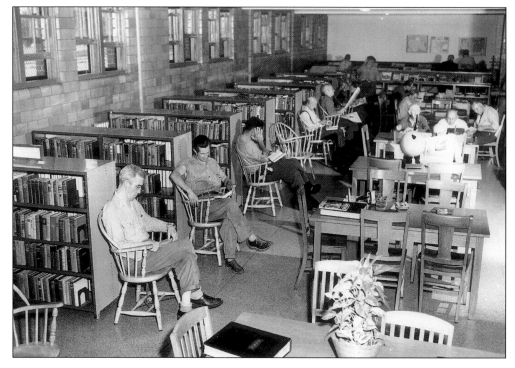

THE ELOISE LIBRARY, 1952. The Eloise branch of the Wayne County Library provided reading materials for patients. The library was located in "N" building or Kelley Hall. The library was founded in 1935 primarily to service the indigent population of "N" building. It had the highest percentage of non-fiction readers of all the County libraries.

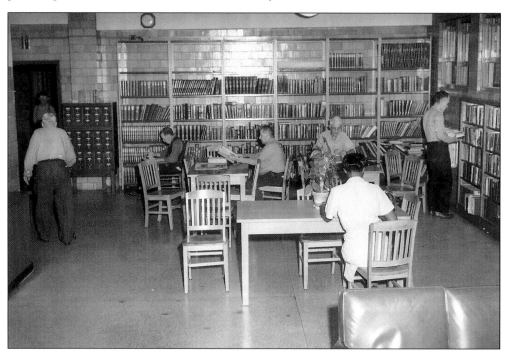

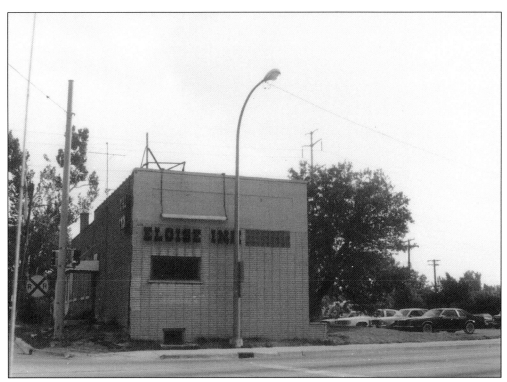

ELOISE INN. Infirmary patients frequented this bar, which was located at the southwest corner of Merriman Road and Michigan Ave. The building was torn down in 2000 and a gas station was erected on this spot.

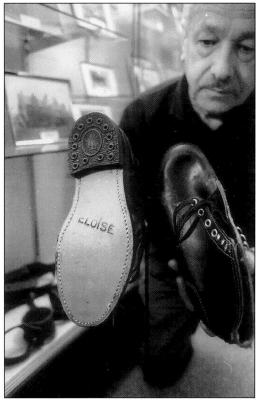

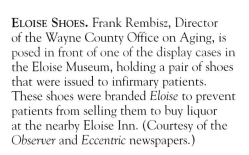

ELOISE SHOES. Frank Rembisz, Director of the Wayne County Office on Aging, is posed in front of one of the display cases in the Eloise Museum, holding a pair of shoes that were issued to infirmary patients. These shoes were branded *Eloise* to prevent patients from selling them to buy liquor at the nearby Eloise Inn. (Courtesy of the *Observer* and *Eccentric* newspapers.)

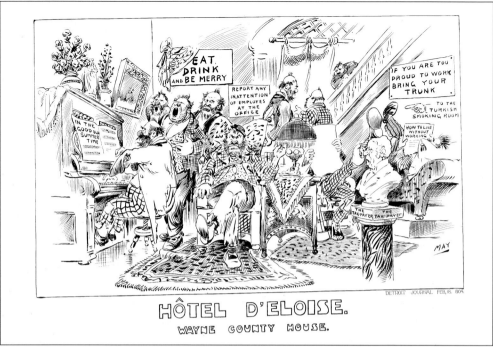

HOTEL D'ELOISE. This cartoon ran on the front page of the *Detroit Journal* February 18, 1904. It was captioned "The Winter Resort at Eloise." The population at Eloise soared when the weather got cold as the indigent population, called wayfarers or tramps in those days, spent their summers on the road and their winters at Eloise.

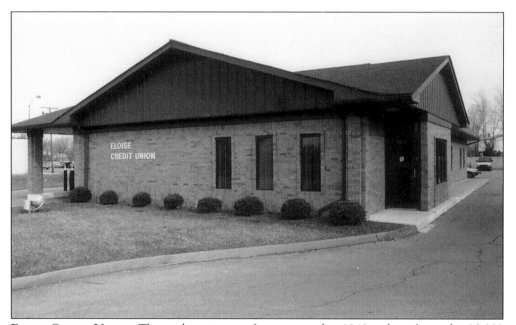

ELOISE CREDIT UNION. The credit union was first organized in 1948 and was located in N-209 in the infirmary building for many years. After the institution closed, a new building was put up on Palmer Road and it is still in business today.

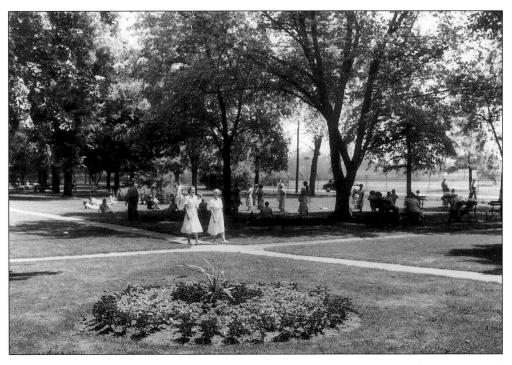

VIEWS OF THE LANDSCAPED GROUNDS OF ELOISE, 1950S. Employees are strolling the grounds and patients are sitting on the many benches that were on the grounds. This was a pleasant way to spend an afternoon when the weather was good.

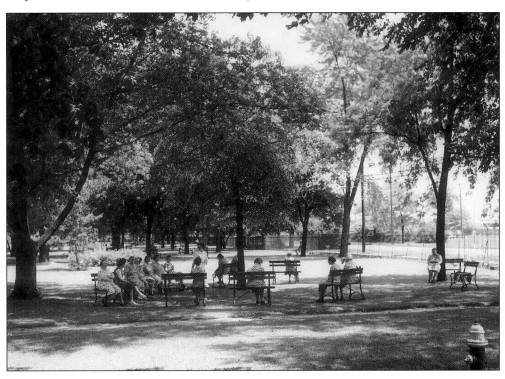

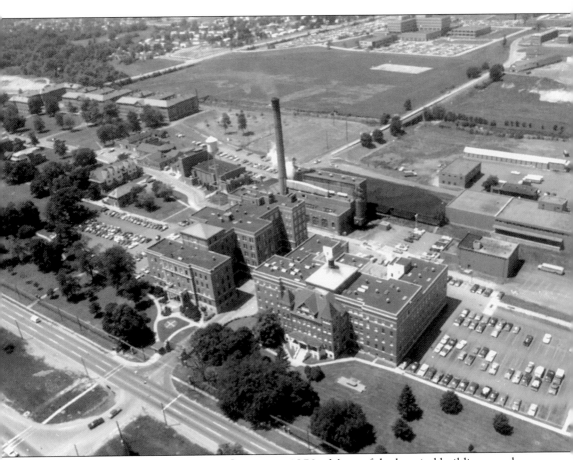

AERIAL VIEW OF THE HOSPITAL GROUNDS, 1970s. Many of the hospital buildings can be seen in this photo taken from Michigan Avenue looking north. "D" Building and the power plant and smokestack are to the left. The large brick building to the right is the William J. Seymour Hospital. "B" Building once stood where the large parking lot is located next to the Seymour Hospital. The Commissary is behind the parking lot, and part of "A" Building can be seen to the far right. In the background is the then new Wayne County General Hospital with "N" Building or Kelley Hall behind it.

Five

FACES OF ELOISE

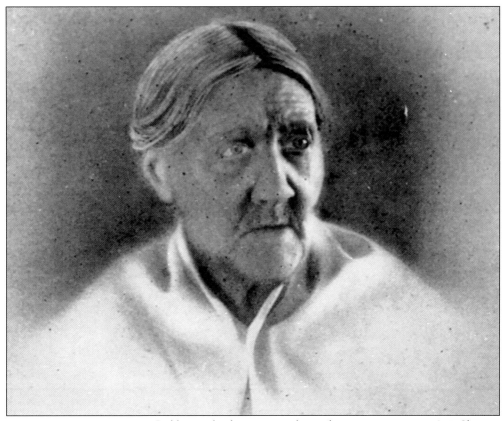

BRIDGET "BIDDY" HUGHES. Biddy was the first person admitted as a *crazy person* in 1841. She was classified as *simple minded* and remained at the County House until her death in 1895. She worked as a culinary assistant serving up a lot of meals in the 54 years she lived at Eloise. Biddy imagined herself to be the sole owner of all she surveyed and kept a careful watch on the tableware.

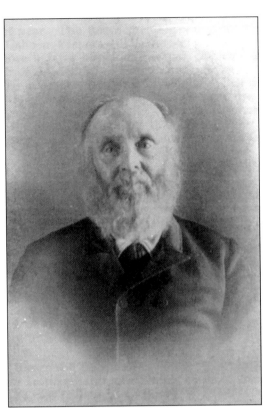

UNCLE JERRY. Jerry Townsend chopped wood for Samuel Torbet. Uncle Jerry also dispensed whiskey at a penny a glass or six for 5¢ for three years at the Black Horse Tavern. He then became a successful farmer, but he fell on hard times and ended up at the County House, maintained in a building erected on the very spot where he had tended bar 60 years before.

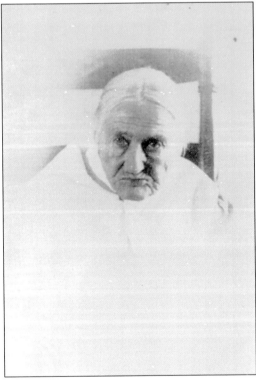

MARY REAGAN. A centenarian inmate of the County House, poor old Mary was described in a Superintendent of the Poor's report as "perched on a chair, with her chin almost on her knees, she smokes a clay pipe the live long day, meditating methods of disagreeableness towards her poverty-condemned sisters."

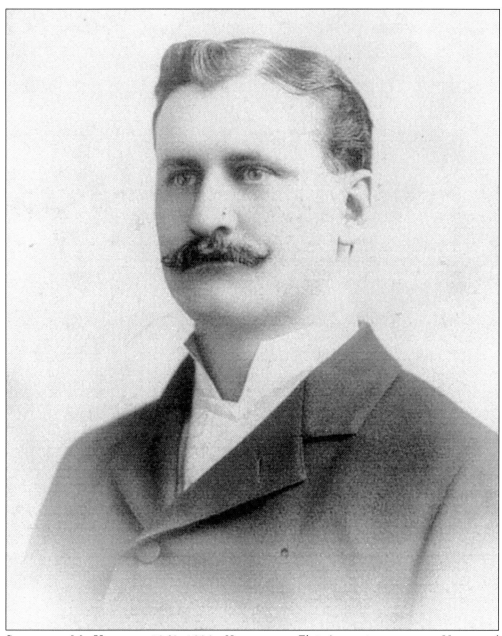

STANISLAS M. KEENAN, 1862–1938. Keenan was Eloise's renaissance man. He started his career as chief bookkeeper at the hospital in 1892 and was also the postmaster and the representative of the Michigan Central Railroad and the American Express Company. He had many other interests including botany, mushrooms, astronomy, history, and electricity. His greatest achievement was as a pioneer in the field of x-rays. The first medical use of x-ray in Michigan in 1896 was to locate a bullet in the foot of an Eloise Hospital patient, and in 1897 Mr. Keenan used an x-ray to show a metallic foreign body in the eye of a patient. This was the first use of an x-ray for this purpose in the U.S. For six years Mr. Keenan did most of the x-rays done in Detroit and Wayne County. He wrote the first book on Eloise titled *History of Eloise* published by Thos. Smith Press in 1913.

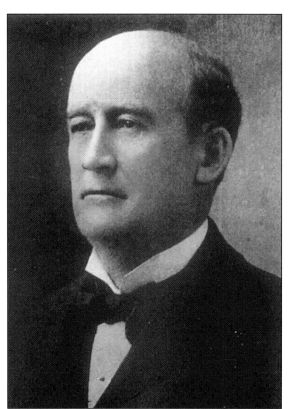

Ebenezer O. Bennett, M.D., First Medical Superintendent, 1881–1900. Prior to the time of his employment, doctors were employed by the year and only were obligated to visit the institution twice a week to provide medical care to the patients. Dr. Bennett was responsible for modernizing the institution, providing better sanitation, and removing the chains, shackles, and dim cells in which the patients had been housed. His son, Joseph E. Bennett, was also a medical superintendent of Eloise.

Janetta D. (Felton) Bennett. She was the wife of Ebenezer O. Bennett and also Matron of the Asylum for 19 years. She maintained a keen interest in the institution after her husband was no longer superintendent.

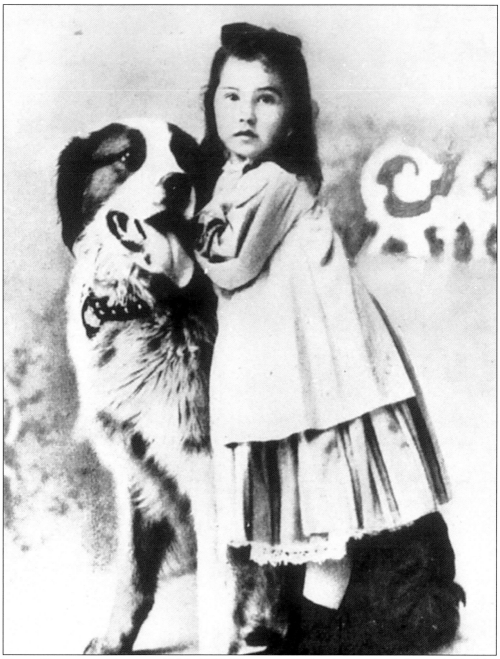

ELOISE DICKERSON DAVOCK, 1888–1982. Eloise was the daughter and only living child of the postmaster of Detroit and the President of the Governing Board of the Wayne County House, Freeman B. Dickerson. Her name was selected by the US Post Office for the name of the post office on the grounds after several other names had been rejected for various reasons. On July 20, 1894, this post office was established under the name of Eloise. The name *Eloise* became a generic term used to designate the complex and all the buildings on it. There are two portraits of Eloise with her St. Bernard companion. One hung in the boardroom of Eloise for many years and later hung in the office of the medical director of Wayne County General Hospital.

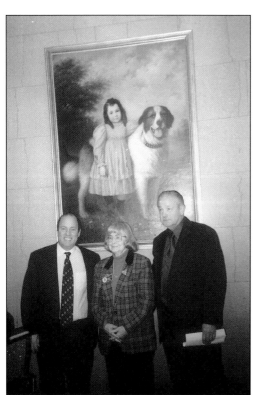

ELOISE RETURNING HOME. In December 2000, at the annual Wayne County General Hospital reunion dinner, Mike Duggan, Deputy County Executive, (left) presented the painting of Eloise, which had been in storage to Commissioner Kay Beard and Frank Rembisz of the Friends of Eloise. It now hangs in the Kay Beard Building.

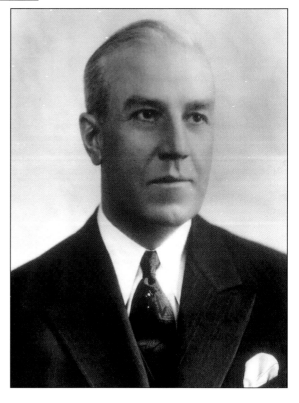

WILLIAM J. SEYMOUR, M.D. Seymour graduated from the Detroit College of Medicine in 1903 and received a L.L.D degree from the University of Detroit in 1933. He was a surgeon and also ran a cancer clinic at Eloise. He was the president of the Public Welfare Commission for ten years. He encouraged the founding of a general hospital to care for the patients at the institution and the general hospital that opened in 1933 was named for him in recognition of his work with the poor. He died in 1945.

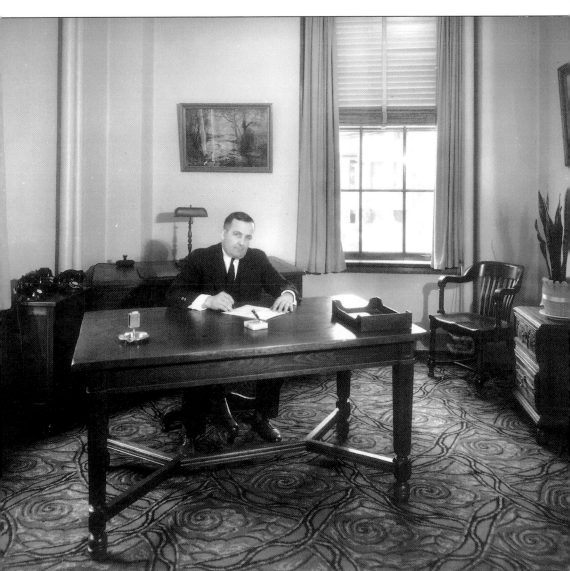

IN CHARGE DURING A RAPID PERIOD OF GROWTH, 1929–1949. Dr. Thomas K. Gruber, General Superintendent of Eloise, is shown in his office in "D" Building. He graduated from Case Western Reserve medical school in 1912 and was an assistant superintendent at Harper Hospital until 1919, when he moved to Rochester, New York. He returned to Detroit in 1921, where he was the superintendent at Receiving Hospital until his appointment at Eloise. Gruber was in charge during the rapid growth of the institution and the construction of several new buildings—"D," "N," "G," "H," "I," "J," "K," "L," "M," and the Auditorium later named the Gruber Auditorium. He guided the institution through the Great Depression when the patient population reached an all-time high. In 1938 Eloise had more than 8,000 patients and 1,800 employees. He died of a heart attack in 1949 at the age of 62, while entertaining friends at his home at Eloise.

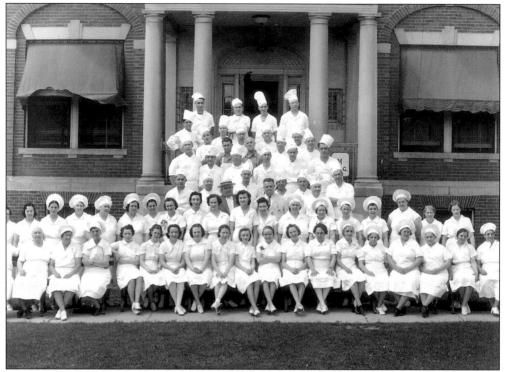

DINING ROOM AND KITCHEN STAFF, JULY 1939. Dr. T.K. Gruber, wearing a straw hat, and Al Hammond the chief steward, wearing a suit, are in the center of a group photo probably taken in front of "M" Building on the day of the annual picnic for the patients. All of the kitchen staff went to the picnic grounds and prepared food for the event. Dishes and silverware and even the bottles of milk had the name *Eloise* on them.

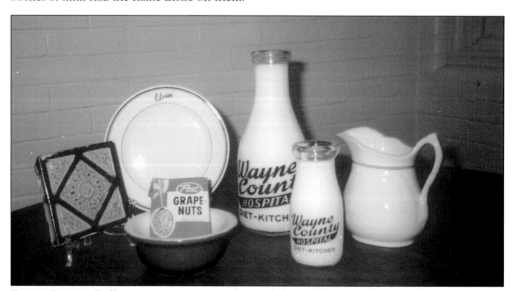

ELOISE DISHES. Different companies manufactured these dishes over the years, but plates, mugs and other items were inscribed *Eloise*. Also shown are the Wayne County Hospital milk bottles and a tile from the "N" Building cafeteria. All are on display in the Eloise museum.

ELOISE BASEBALL TEAM, 1940.
Dr. Walter Hale Squires and his son,
Joseph Robert Squires, proudly represent
the Eloise baseball team. Dr. Squires
was the psychiatrist in charge of the
male division of the psychiatric services.
Joseph Robert, known as Bob, and his
sister, Betty, were born and raised on
the grounds.

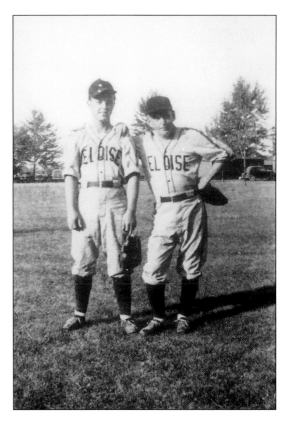

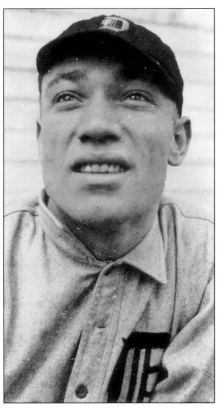

MARTY KAVANAGH, 1914. Martin Joseph
Kavanagh (1891–1960) was one of several
professional baseball players who died at Eloise. His
major league debut was April 18, 1914, as a Detroit
Tiger. He played for the Tigers in 1915 and part of
1916, and then played for the Cleveland Indians.
On September 24, 1918, while a utility infielder for
the Cleveland Indians, he hit the first pinch-hit
grand-slam home run in the American League.
The ball rolled through a hole in the fence and
everyone scored. (Courtesy of the Burton Historical
Collection of the Detroit Public Library.)

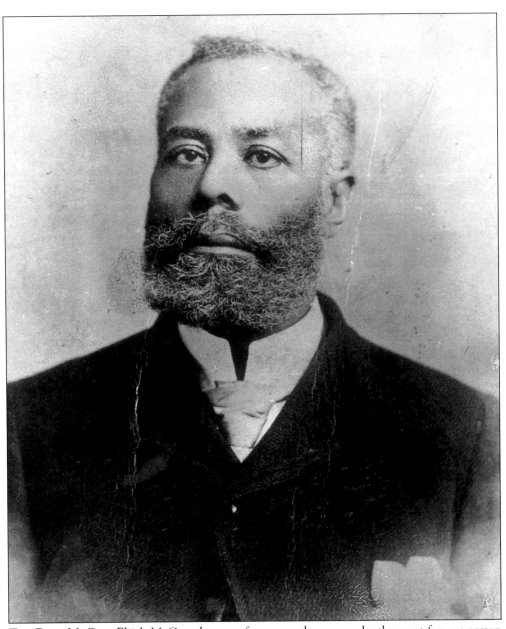

THE REAL McCOY. Elijah McCoy, the son of runaway slaves, may be the most famous person treated at Eloise. McCoy was born in Canada in 1844, and he went to school in Scotland where he served an apprenticeship in mechanical engineering. Unable to get work in that field, he went to work as a brakeman and fireman on trains running between Detroit and Ann Arbor. He started designing improvements in lubricating systems for trains that were later adapted for use on other machinery. People came from all over the world to make sure they were getting "The Real McCoy." This became an American expression meaning the real thing. McCoy fell on hard times and ended up as a patient in Eloise suffering from senile dementia and hypertension. He died in the Eloise Infirmary October 10, 1929. He was buried as a pauper in the Eloise cemetery, but friends later raised funds to have his body moved to a site in Detroit Memorial Park. (Courtesy of the Burton Historical Collection of the Detroit Public Library.)

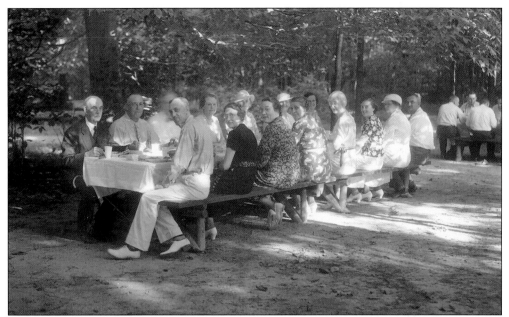

STAFF PICNIC, 1930S. Bill Hudson, the head gardener, is the first person on the right side of the picnic bench. John Near, a member of the hospital board, is on the other side of the table.

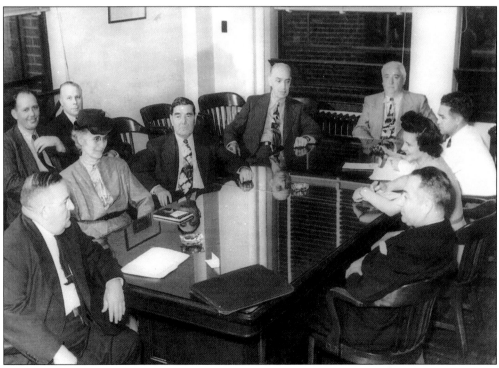

MEETING OF THE HOSPITAL BOARD, 1940S. Seated around the table are, from the front left: Dr. Thomas K. Gruber, Adelia D. Starrett, James H. Garlick, Dr. Edward F. Fisher, Frank E. Kelley, two unidentified people, and Monroe Lake. Kelley Hall or "N" Building was named after Frank E. Kelley, who served on the governing board of Eloise for many years.

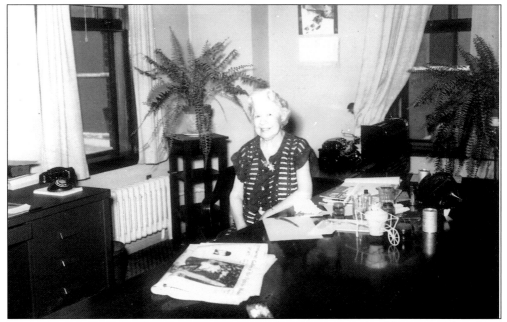

FIRST WAYNE COUNTY RETIREE, 1945. Mrs. Alice B. Keenan, bookkeeper at the Eloise Hospital for 52 years, is pictured at her desk. She was the first to file for an application for retirement under the provisions of the Wayne County Employees Retirement System. She was the daughter of Joseph Waltz, founder of Waltz, Michigan, and the wife of Stanislas M. Keenan, the chief bookkeeper. They lived on the Eloise grounds.

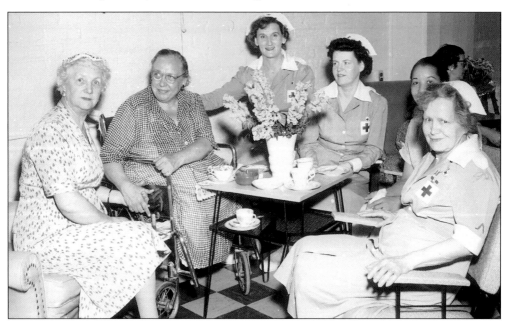

SHARING SOME COFFEE AND CONVERSATION, 1950S. This photo shows Eloise staff and volunteers with a patient. From left to right, they are: Mrs. Margaret C. Doyle, Hospital Board Chairman, Helen Brown, a patient, (in wheelchair), two unidentified Gray Ladies, Miss Smith, a music therapist, Miss Willis, Head Nurse, and Mrs. Hall, a Gray Lady.

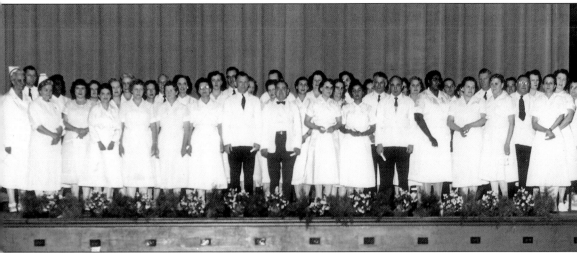

EMPLOYEE AWARDS, 1950S. The stage of the Gruber Auditorium is full of employees, probably attendants, who are holding certificates. At the far left are two registered nurses.

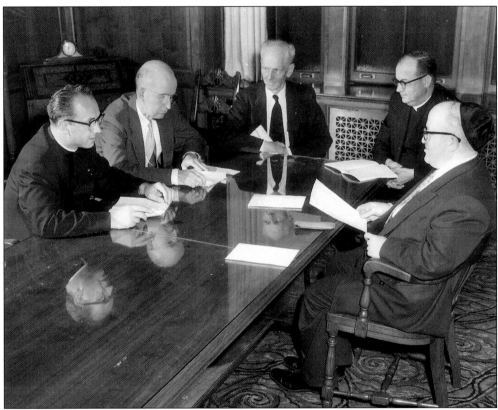

HOSPITAL CHAPLAINS, 1952. Seated in the hospital board room are, from left to right: Rev. Leonard Zak, Catholic Chaplain, Rev. R.A.N. Wilson Jr., Protestant Chaplain, Rev. H.S. Quitmeyer, Lutheran Chaplain, Rev. Edwin S. Milka, Catholic Chaplain, and Rabbi M. Wahlgelernter. They provided for the spiritual needs of the patients and employees and some lived on the grounds.

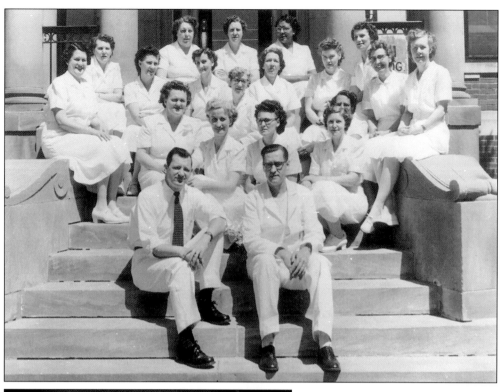

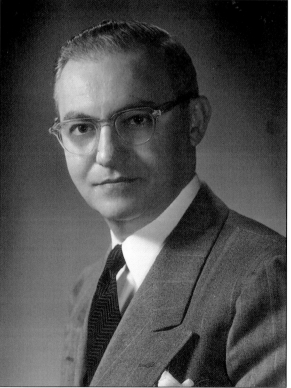

EDUCATION AT ELOISE, 1954. In this photo of the Practical Nurse class taken on the steps of "L" or "M" Building, Director of Nurses John Wisniewski is in the front left. The hospital also ran its own x-ray technologist school for many years. The hospital was used for training and affiliations with several local universities and colleges such as the medical schools at Wayne State and the University of Michigan. It was also affiliated with Henry Ford Community College, Schoolcraft Community College, and Madonna College's programs in nursing.

SYLVESTER E. GOULD, M.D. Sylvester E. Gould was the chief pathologist for the William J. Seymour Hospital and in 1952 did research on the cause and cures of pork trichinosis. He also wrote "The Story of Eloise and Wayne County General Hospital" for the *Detroit Medical News* in 1962. (Photo by Paul Gach.)

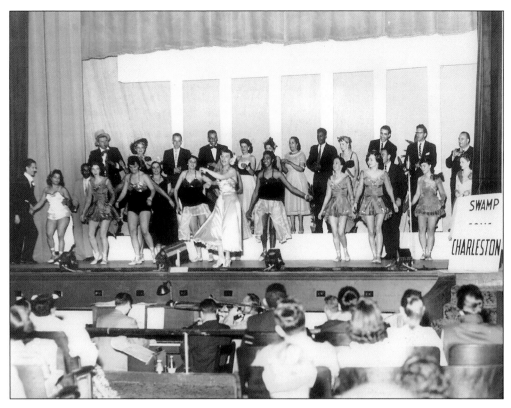

EMPLOYEE PERFORMANCE, 1950S. These employees are putting on a performance for friends, family and fellow employees in the Gruber Auditorium. Note the band in the orchestra pit.

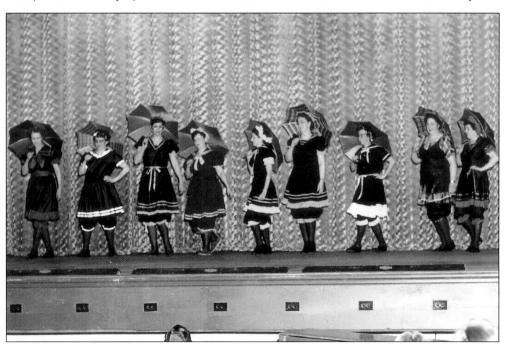

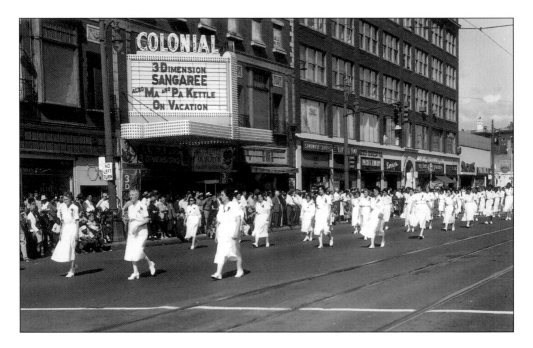

Marching in the Labor Day Parade, 1953. Eloise employees won several awards for being the best dressed in the annual Labor Day parades held in downtown Detroit. The parade is shown in front of the Colonial Theater in the first photo and at Woodward and Montcalm in the second.

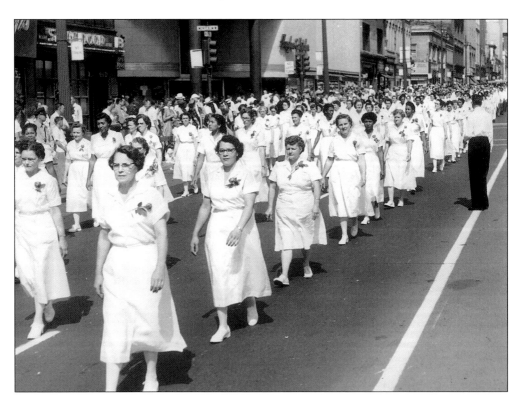

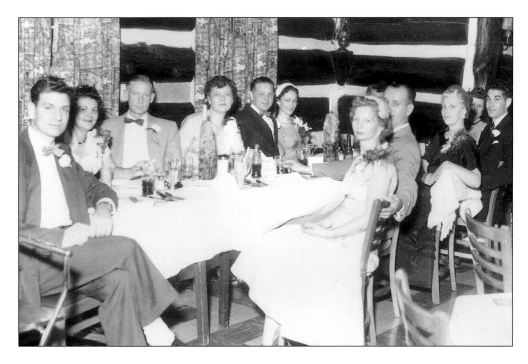

EMPLOYEE PARTIES, 1950S. The first group of unidentified employees was attending a dinner party. The second group is having a picnic in a park complete with dancing girls and a fortuneteller.

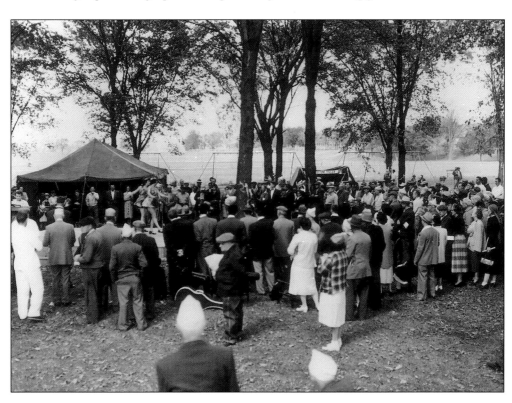

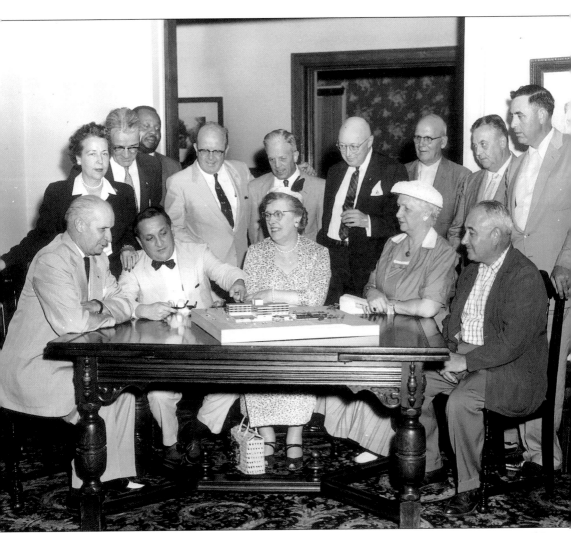

HOSPITAL OFFICIALS LOOKING OVER MODEL OF PROPOSED NEW GENERAL HOSPITAL, 1957.
In this photo taken by M. Sandy Blakeman in 1957, the participants are viewing a model of the new general hospital. They are, from left to right: (seated) Mayor of Ecorse, William W. Voisine, Chairman, Wayne County General Hospital Committee of Board of Supervisors; Dr. S.D. Jacobson, Hospital Superintendent; Mrs. Margaret Abernethy, Hospital Board member; Mrs. Margaret C. Doyle, Chairman of the Hospital Board, and Mr. Monroe Lake, Hospital Board member; (standing) Mrs. Blanche Parent Wise, Mr. Andrew S. McFarlane, Mr. Alexander Fuller, Mr. Martin Fleming, Mr. Roy R. Lindsay, Dr. Robert V. Walker, Mr. Chase Stottlemyer, Mr. Francis H. Bailey, and Mr. Terry L. Trout. All are members of the Hospital Committee of the Board of Supervisors except for Mr. Fleming.

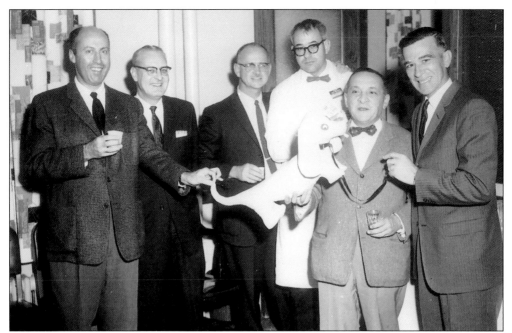

HOSPITAL ADMINISTRATORS, 1960S. They are, from left to right: Marvin Lawrence, Hugh Armbruster, Les Aspinall, Hershel Wells, M.D., General Superintendent of Wayne County General Hospital and Long Term Care Facility from May 24, 1965 to March 4, 1974, Samuel Jacobson, M.D., holding the dachshund, and Robert Mitrovich.

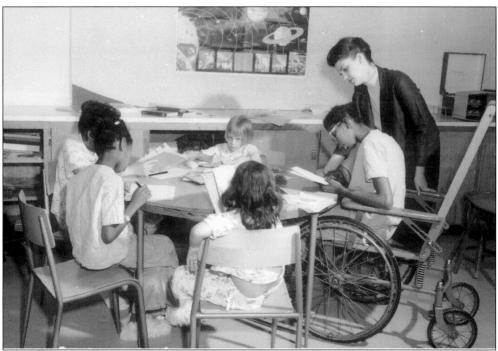

CLASSES IN THE PEDIATRIC PLAYROOM, 1965. These children are being taught their lessons by a visiting teacher in the playroom on 5 North in the General Hospital.

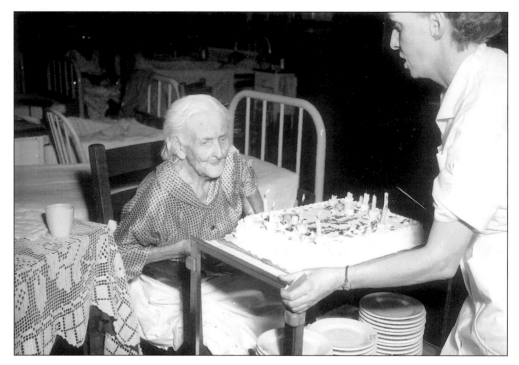

CELEBRATING A BIRTHDAY IN "N" BUILDING, 1960S. A birthday was an occasion for celebration and the bakery produced cakes for resident's birthdays. Many of the residents in the infirmary division were of advanced age. All the patients joined in the celebration, as evidenced by the stack of plates on the cart.

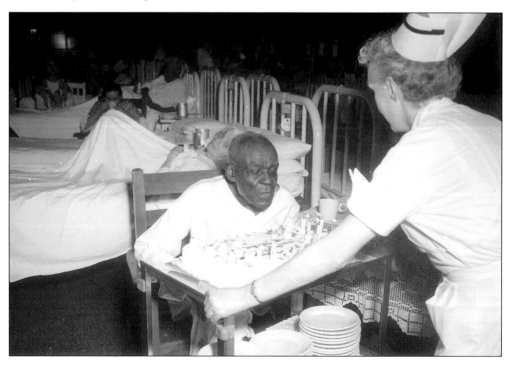

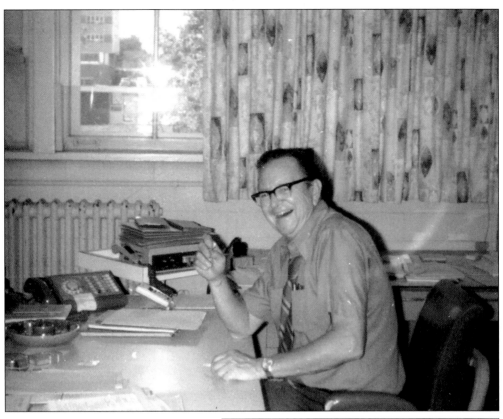

ALVIN C. CLARK, 1920–1996.
Clark, shown here in a lighter
moment in his office in "N" Building,
was a pharmacist by profession, but
was the head of hospital personnel
and an Eloise historian. He wrote
the second book on Eloise in 1982
titled A History of the Wayne County
Infirmary, Psychiatric, and General
Hospital Complex at Eloise, Michigan.

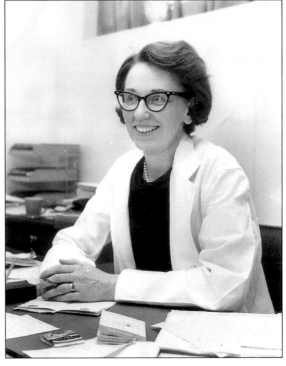

EMMA J. CONKLIN, M.D. Dr. Conklin
had a long association with Eloise as
a member of the medical staff from
1950 on. She was the Executive
Administrator of the General Hospital
from 1978 until the hospital closed
in 1984.

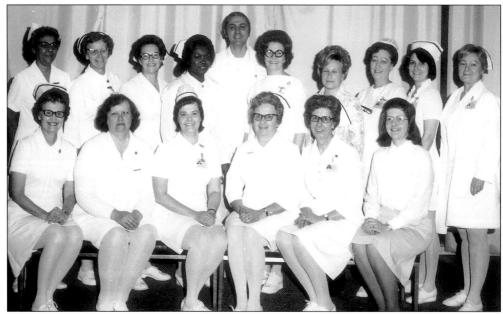

GENERAL HOSPITAL NURSING OFFICE STAFF, 1976. The staff is, from left to right: (front row, seated) Minton Sicklesteel, R.N., Barbara Bergman, R.N., Helen White, R.N., Mary Horbal, R.N., Rita Gac Murdock, R.N., and Phyllis Stamoran; (back row) Nancy Landingham, R.N., Roselyn M. Beller, R.N., Geraldine Fitzpatrick, R.N., Bertha Crossley, R.N., Orville Tews, R.N., Director of Nurses, Juanita Brannock, R.N., Jean Reeves, Sue DeBaldo, R.N., Sue Lund, R.N., and Yolan Mickel, R.N.

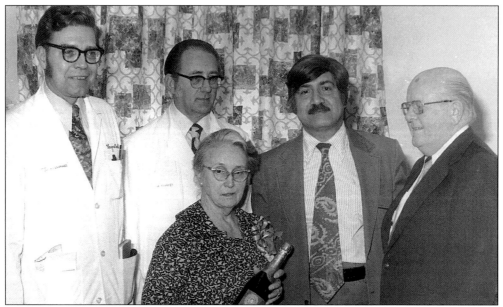

HAPPY OCCASION, 1970S. Psychiatrist Edward Missavage; Merlin C. Townley, Director of the Psychiatric Division; psychiatrist Morteza Minui; and Martin Fleming, member of the Wayne County Board of County Institutions, are shown honoring Natalia Janecki (holding bottle of champagne) on the occasion of her retirement.

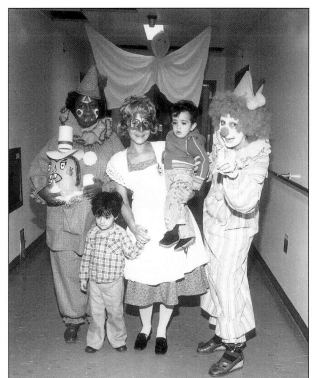

DRESSED UP FOR HALLOWEEN, 1970S. Staff members of the O.B./GYN and Pediatric Clinics are wearing costumes for Halloween. The O.B./GYN Clinic was located in the Walter P. Reuther Long Term Care facility at that time.

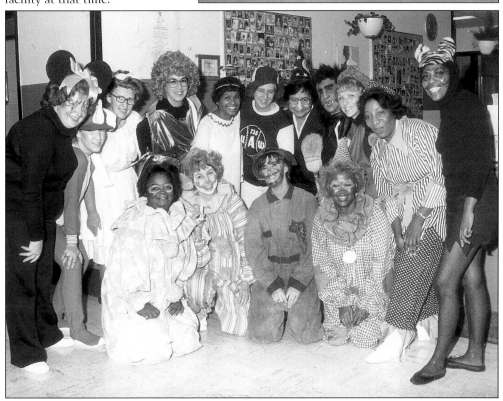

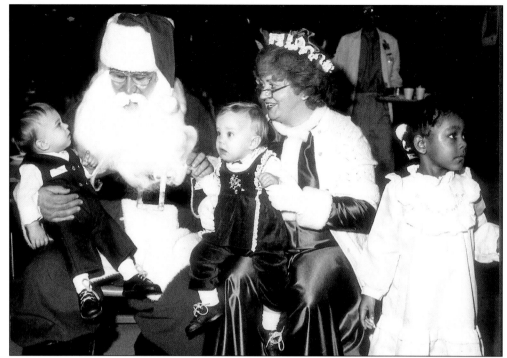

SANTA AND MRS. CLAUS, 1970S. Dr. Steve Koeff, a pediatrician, and Sandra Stoecklein, a registered nurse, hold graduates of the hospital's neonatal intensive care unit. An annual holiday reunion was held for all the children who had been born at Wayne County General Hospital and were little patients in this unit.

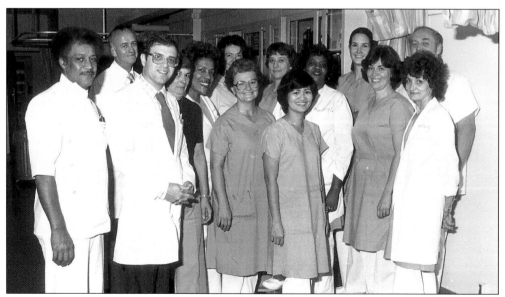

SMILING STAFF OF THE KIDNEY UNIT, C. 1980. These people were the pioneers in kidney dialysis in Michigan. Dr. Gerald A. Rigg is at the left in the second row and Patsy Janes, R.N., Head Nurse, is at the far right in this group photo of the kidney unit staff. Dr. Paul Kissner is second to the left in the front row.

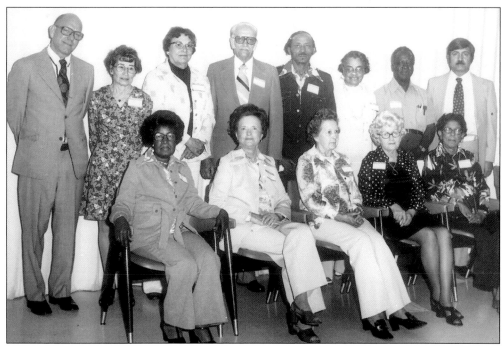

RETIREE LUNCHEON, 1976. Hospital retirees—all sitting in the front row, J. Juanita Jackson, Mary Foley, Mary Nichols, Eleanor Rosenkranz, and Frances Lovejoy—were feted at a luncheon celebrating their retirement. In the back row are James McGlincy, Vernice M. Parrish, Marie H. Grimoldby, Walter Kasten, Adolphus Strother, Annie Stewart, John C. Norman, and Morteza Minui, M.D.

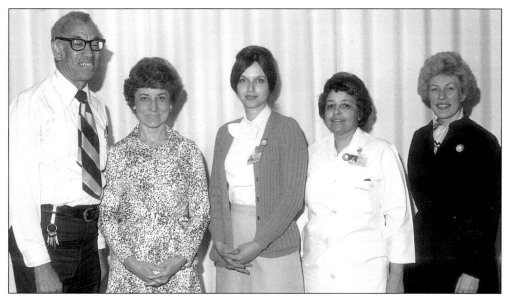

HOSPITAL EMPLOYEES, 1970S. Phelmon Saunders, supervisor of the print shop, Marilyn Madlinger, a secretary in administration, Penelope Foley, R.N., nursing services, Winnie Byrd, hospital laboratory, and Nancy Rowles, supervisor of admitting and information, pose for the camera.

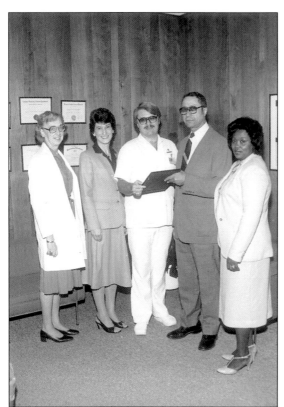

EMPLOYEES OF THE MONTH, 1980S. Every month outstanding employees were presented with awards for their service to the hospital. Dr. E.J. Conklin, Patricia Ibbotson, and Bertha Crossley, watch as Dr. Lawrence S. Lackey, vice chairman of the hospital board, presents the award to Gary Curry, R.N. In the second photo Walter Rosiek and Joe Magda, watch as Michael Bradley, chairman of the hospital board, presents the award to Vinai Sikka.

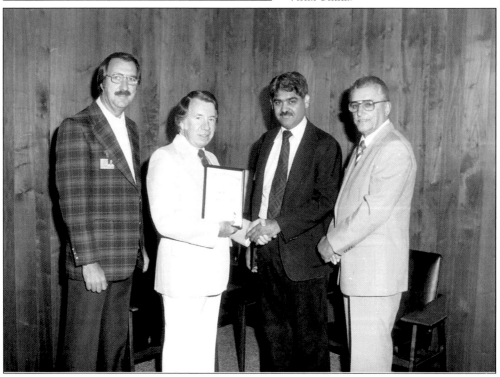

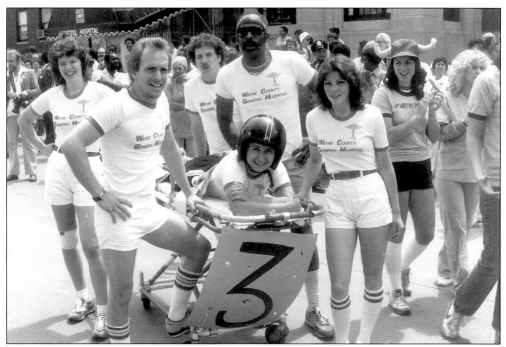

GREAT STRETCHER RACE, 1982. Jane Owens, David Buckley, Pat DePonio, Chester Godley, and Patti Kukula-Chylinski with "patient" Sue Lund, on the stretcher in front of Hutzel Hospital. Hutzel Hospital sponsored and won the event that year.

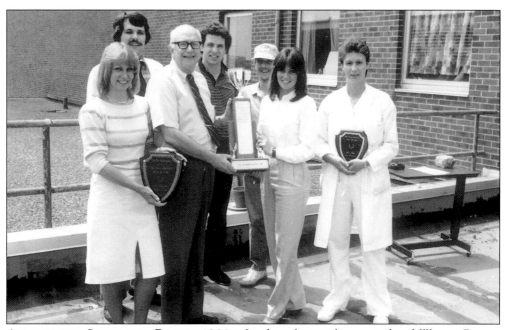

AWARDS FOR STRETCHER RACES, 1980s. In this photo taken outside of Wayne County General Hospital, Nancy Roggero, Chris Kosma, Pat DePonio, David Buckley (wearing hat), Leonard Forster, assistant to the executive administrator, Patti Kukula-Chylinski, and Kim Yesh are holding awards.

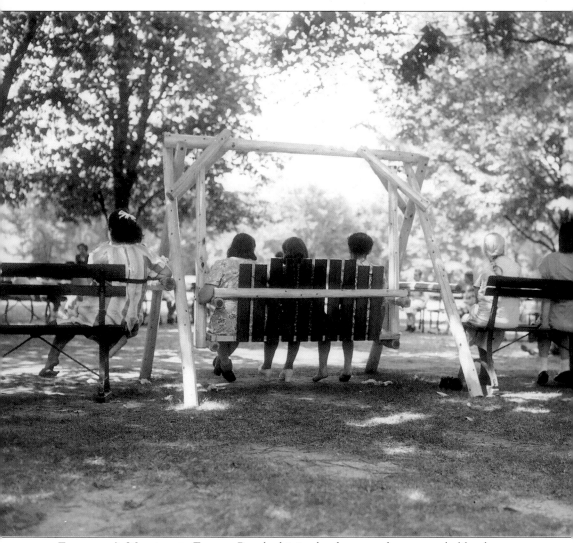

EVERYONE'S MEMORY OF ELOISE. People driving by the grounds saw people like these women, photographed in 1952, sitting on the swings and benches that faced Michigan Avenue. An iron fence had been put up in 1917 that enclosed the grounds. Many curiosity seekers used to come out to Eloise on Sundays and holidays. They trampled over the lawns and gardens, had picnic lunches and played baseball. The fence was put up not to keep the patients in as much as it was to keep the public out. The gates to the new fence were closed on weekends, and permission was required to enter the grounds. After the fence was put up, these patients were all that most of the public saw of Eloise. In the minds of many people Eloise was a place apart, a place of last resort for the mentally ill, the poor, the aged, and the infirm.